ADRIAN PATTERSON DDS.
3204 SHORTRIDGE LANE
MITCHELLVILLE, MD 20721

Manual of CUTANEOUS LASER TECHNIQUES

Manual of Cutaneous Laser Techniques

Tina S. Alster, MD

Director, Washington Institute of Dermatologic
  Laser Surgery
Clinical Assistant Professor, Georgetown
  University Medical Center
Washington, DC
Lecturer, Harvard Medical School
Boston, Massachusetts

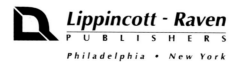

Lippincott - Raven
P U B L I S H E R S
Philadelphia • New York

Acquisitions Editor: Richard Winters
Coordinating Editorial Assistant: Erin O'Connor
Project Editor: Grace R. Caputo
Production Manager: Caren Erlichman
Production Coordinator: David Yurkovich
Design Coordinator: Kathy Kelley-Luedtke
Indexer: Lynne Mahan
Compositor: Maryland Composition
Printer: Quebecor/Kingsport

Library of Congress Cataloging-in-Publication Data
Alster, Tina S.
    Manual of cutaneous laser techniques/Tina S. Alster.
        p.   cm.
    Includes bibliographical references and index.
    ISBN 0-397-58429-6 (alk. paper)
    1. Skin—Laser surgery—Handbooks, manuals, etc.   I. Title.
    [DNLM: 1. Laser Surgery—methods.   2. Skin Diseases—surgery.   WO
511 A463, 1997]
RL120.L37A45   1997
617.4′77059—dc21
DNLM/DLC
for Library of Congress   96-37985
                                                              CIP

Care has been taken to confirm the accuracy of the information presented and to describe generally accepted practices. However, the authors, editors, and publisher are not responsible for errors or omissions or for any consequences from application of the information in this book and make no warranty, express or implied, with respect to the contents of the publication.

The authors, editors, and publisher have exerted every effort to ensure that drug selection and dosage set forth in this text are in accordance with current recommendations and practice at the time of publication. However, in view of ongoing research, changes in government regulations, and the constant flow of information relating to drug therapy and drug reactions, the reader is urged to check the package insert for each drug for any change in indications and dosage and for added warnings and precautions. This is particularly important when the recommended agent is a new or infrequently employed drug.

Some drugs and medical devices presented in this publication have Food and Drug Administration (FDA) clearance for limited use in restricted research settings. It is the responsibility of the health care provider to ascertain the FDA status of each drug or device planned for use in their clinical practice.

9   8   7   6   5   4   3   2   1

ACKNOWLEDGMENTS

During the course of my formal education and postgraduate training, I had the great fortune to be influenced by a number of exceptional physicians. A formal acknowledgment goes to the following, who, probably unknowingly, have served as my mentors and role models: Claude Burton, MD, Leonard Dzubow, MD, Richard Edelson, MD, Peter Heald, MD, Steven Kohn, MD, Leonard Milstone, MD, Elise Olsen, MD, Sheldon Pinnell, MD, and Sheldon Pollack, MD.

My laser colleagues—notably Rox Anderson, MD, Kenneth Arndt, MD, Brian Biesman, MD, Jeffrey Dover, MD, Richard Fitzpatrick, MD, Jerome Garden, MD, Roy Geronemus, MD, David Goldberg, MD, Mitchel Goldman, MD, Joop Grevelink, MD, George Hruza, MD, Arielle Kauvar, MD, Suzanne Kilmer, MD, Gary Lask, MD, Nicholas Lowe, MD, Harvey Lui, MD, John Ratz, MD, Oon Tian Tan, MD, Walter Unger, MD, and Ronald Wheeland, MD—have all not only made valuable scientific contributions but have willingly shared their insights and knowledge with me. I extend my sincere gratitude to them for their honesty, criticisms, and support.

The input of fellows and students who continue to ask me questions that prompt further inquiry into this ever-expanding science also cannot be underestimated. I thank them as well as my patients, who honor me with their trust and optimism.

A special acknowledgment goes to my staff—especially Georgina Eva, Karin Formica, RN, Louisa Huband, Christopher Nanni, MD, Michael Stokes, and Tina West, MD—who tolerated my more harried moments and assisted in the compilation of data needed to complete the final manuscript. An individual word of thanks goes to my editor, Richard Winters, who first conceived of and proposed the concept for this book.

Finally, my most heartfelt appreciation goes to my husband, Ambassador Paul Frazer, whose endless support and encouragement helped me to realize this endeavor. This book is dedicated to him and our newborn son, Nicholas.

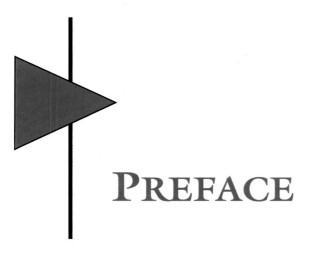

PREFACE

"Don't learn the tricks of the trade. Learn the trade."
—*Anonymous*

No words ring as true as these when the subject of cutaneous laser surgery is raised. This extraordinary technology has truly revolutionized the practice of dermatology, leading to innovative treatments for a host of skin conditions that only a few years ago were regarded as all but intractable. The advances have occurred so rapidly and with such dazzling effect that it sometimes seems they are a result of a conjurer's tricks. Yet, like any other surgical instrument, a laser is merely a tool. And those who wield it are not magicians, but craftsmen, practicing a unique trade that demands careful study.

My own apprenticeship began a decade ago, during my dermatology residency at Yale. A 44-year-old woman sought my help for the treatment of one of the most psychologically devastating of all skin conditions. A large, dark port-wine stain—raised and colored an angry purplish red—covered half her face. It extended up her neck, over her chin, and across her left cheek all the way into her ear. My patient told a typically heart-rending tale. She wept as she recounted the stares she had endured all her life, the taunts she had heard as a child, the discrimination she had encountered in the workplace, and the agonizing self-consciousness she had felt in even her closest personal relationships. Despite it all, she had persevered to pursue a successful career in advertising, to marry, and to have a child. Yet this seemingly assured professional woman was so agonizingly embarrassed by her disfigurement that neither her friends or colleagues nor even her husband or teenage son had ever seen her face without its customary heavy covering of camouflage makeup.

The patient had been referred to me because of my special interest in cosmetic dermatology. But that day I had to tell her the same thing she had heard from every other doctor she had ever seen: I knew of nothing that could be done to improve the appearance of her birthmark without creating an equally disfiguring scar. At the time, the use of cutaneous lasers was limited to a few innovative physicians and a handful of research facilities. When I went into the library to explore the possibility of using a laser on this woman's port-wine stain, I found one up-to-date clinical article on the subject.

Following that lead ultimately led me to pursue a laser fellowship under the tutelage of Dr. Oon Tian Tan in Boston. There, I was extremely fortunate to participate in many of the original clinical investigations using modern dermatologic lasers and to practice this infant technology in one of the few medical facilities in the world where it was then being regularly employed. A little more than a year after my patient left the Yale clinic in tears, I was able to begin a series of treatments that eventually removed her birthmark with barely a trace, giving her the smooth unmarred complexion she had yearned for since childhood.

Today, thousands of adults who grew up believing they were literally marked for life have had disfiguring birthmarks either erased or reduced into virtual insignificance through laser surgery. Infants who enter the world with these once lifelong malformations can now grow up never conscious of having had them. The groundbreaking laser that made this modern medical miracle possible is now widely used to treat other vascular lesions, such as hemangiomas and telangiectasias. Moreover, we now have lasers that can smooth a complexion pitted by acne or chickenpox scars or remove solar lentigines and café-au-lait macules. Others can erase tattoos or restore severely burned or scarred skin to a more normal appearance.

Most recently, high-energy, pulsed or scanned carbon dioxide lasers that literally vaporize skin in a layer-by-layer fashion have become the most feverishly hyped weapons in the war on photodamaged skin. So much media attention has been focused on their capacity to bloodlessly peel away wrinkles that thousands of patients have swarmed into doctors' offices seeking laser firepower to turn back the clocks on their aging faces.

Thousands of physicians are now adding cosmetic lasers to their practices. Ongoing laser research and the publication of findings in medical journals have increased exponentially. One can hardly escape the blitz of magazine articles and television news stories on the miracles of laser surgery.

Unfortunately, the increasingly widespread availability of cosmetic laser therapy coupled with the attendant publicity has created extraordinary, often unrealistic expectations. Many patients really do believe that lasers are indeed magic wands, capable of restoring their skin to the flawless perfection of infancy. And even skeptical physicians can become so captivated by the amazing potential of these surgical tools that they may lose sight of their limitations and their demands. The truth, of course, is that cosmetic lasers are not a panacea for all dermatologic ills. And while laser surgery is, on the whole, less painful and risky than many of the techniques it has replaced, it is still surgery, with the potential complications that attend any surgical procedure.

Manual of Cutaneous Laser Techniques was written to give practitioners new to the field or those with early laser experience who are considering expanding their laser horizons a realistic look at the various lasers available and to help practitioners become comfortable with their use. It presents a review of the lasers used to treat a variety of dermatologic lesions. In addition, it gives specific guidelines on patient preparation, intraoperative set-up, and laser treatment protocols, as well as postoperative patient management. I hope it will be an aid in learning the laser trade, rather than merely its tricks.

Tina S. Alster, MD

CONTENTS

Manual of

CUTANEOUS
LASER
TECHNIQUES

Manual of Cutaneous Laser Techniques, by Tina S. Alster.
Lippincott–Raven Publishers, Philadelphia © 1997.

CHAPTER 1

GETTING STARTED: SETTING UP A LASER PRACTICE

Patient Considerations ► *Office or Facility Considerations* ► *Training Considerations* ► *Market Considerations* ► *Financial Considerations* ► *Laser Considerations* ► *Marketing Your New Laser*

Establishing a laser practice is no easy task, so the decision to enter into this exciting field should be carefully studied. Numerous dermatologic lasers are available for lease or purchase: many of them can treat the same type of lesion, but no one laser can treat all kinds of cutaneous lesions. The variety of technology includes pulsed dye systems, quality-switched (Q-switched or QS) systems, and continuous wave (CW) systems. You should become familiar with the different technologies available to make an informed decision about which particular laser is suitable for your practice. Laser salespersons and promotional brochures cannot provide the complete picture about a particular laser's clinical suitability. The old adage, "you get what you pay for," comes to mind whenever I hear a salesperson extol the virtues and superior benefits of a single laser that can treat everything from a simple telangiectasia to a complex tattoo. In fact, more than one kind of laser is often needed to treat a single lesion, such as a multicolored tattoo. So, it is imperative that we, as physicians and consumers, study the technology closely so that the appropriate array of lasers is used for different presenting lesions.

Before actually selecting the laser or lasers you need, it is necessary that you assess several factors pertaining to your practice (Table 1-1).

TABLE 1-1. EVALUATING YOUR PRACTICE

Patient Profile	Office Setup	Laser Training	Local Factors	Financial Considerations
Pediatric vs adult Birthmark vs cosmetic Self-pay vs insurance	Physical requirements • Correct voltage • Separate room Anesthesia supplies Safety factors Other equipment (smoke evacuator)	Physician Ancillary medical staff Office staff	Competing MDs or laser centers Referral network Community-at-large	Lease or buy? Associated expenses • Maintenance contract • Laser disposables (dye cartridges)

▶ Patient Considerations

The first step in determining whether the addition of a laser is appropriate is a careful review of your patient profile. Do you primarily see pediatric or adult patients or an even mix of both? Most pediatric patients present for treatment of birthmarks (port-wine stain, hemangioma, or café-au-lait spot), whereas adult patients typically present with lesions consistent with photodamage (solar lentigines, poikiloderma, rhytides). You probably already have a subset of patients who have failed more traditional forms of treatment, such as cryotherapy and electrodesiccation, for such lesions as lentigines and telangiectasias who now desire more selective or definitive laser treatment. Thus, your patient profile determines which laser or lasers would be appropriate for your practice.

If most of your patients are self-payors rather than dependent on insurance coverage (or if you are intending to change your practice management so that it is that way), then the addition of a laser to your practice will pose no problems. On the other hand, you will need to inform your patients who are covered by Medicare, managed care plans, or other insurance policies that most of these plans exclude laser treatment coverage simply on cosmetic grounds. Certainly, insurance reimbursement for laser treatment of extensive or devastating lesions, such as port-wine stains, café-au-lait birthmarks, and scars, may be approved on an individual basis. Even those patients who would normally file for insurance coverage may elect to become self-payors if they believe that the laser surgery would be worthwhile and if they have the monetary resources.

▶ Office or Facility Considerations

Your office setup should also be given consideration when planning to add a laser. Because lasers and their corresponding accessories (eg, smoke evacuators) take up space, at least one extra room in which to house the laser or lasers will be needed. Special electrical and water requirements are necessary for some lasers. Proper lighting for the laser procedure may require the installation of extra operating lights. Because of excessive heat production from the operation of the lasers, adequate ventilation in the room should be ascertained. In addition, the risk of

TABLE 1-2. **SAFETY PROCEDURE CHECKLIST**

Issue	Policy
Flammability	Fire extinquisher
	Water and wet cloths
	Nonreflective instruments
	No alcohol preparations
	Keep laser in "standby" when not in use
Ocular safety	Appropriate eyewear without reflective metal
Electrical hazards	Dedicated outlets for laser use
	No extension cords
	No defects in laser cord
	No water or other solutions near laser
Controlled access to laser suite	Warning and danger signs posted on doors
	Opaque material on windows
	Laser keys locked when not in use
Laser plume	Smoke evacuator with clean filter and tubing
	Laser masks

transmission of laser light through glass requires that any windows existing in the treatment room be covered with opaque material. Other safety considerations, such as proper storage and placement of anesthetic materials, including oxygen, should be thoroughly reviewed so that Occupational Health and Safety Administration (OSHA) requirements are met. Although OSHA does not regulate the use of lasers in health care, it acts as an advocate for workers on the job site. Thus, the development of a safety program that functions in compliance with OSHA's regulations should be taken seriously. That means that the physical laser facility must comply with safety standards and that all employees should be well-versed in the safety policies and procedures outlined for the office (Table 1-2).

▶ Training Considerations

No national standards or criteria exist for laser training. No boards or examinations are required for either physicians or nurses to become certified in laser surgery. As such, educational criteria and terms for credentialing physicians, nurses, and other health care workers should be established individually by each office or medical facility, based on the broad recommendations of such professional organizations as the American Academy of Dermatology and the American Society for Laser Medicine and Surgery. At a minimum, physicians should complete a formal course in laser surgery that covers laser physics, laser safety and operation, indications and contraindications for laser surgery, and hands-on laser experience under competent supervision. Evidence of documented clinical laser experience may be obtained after a preceptorship. Nurses and ancillary medical staff should receive initial and continuing education that focuses on safety issues, patient education, and intraoperative and postoperative documentation. This can be accomplished by attending physician or nursing seminars at national laser surgery meetings, such as the American Society for Laser Medicine and Surgery, which has established criteria for laser nursing practice standards. Because the laser field is growing so rapidly, it is imperative that practitioners not only receive initial training, but also continue to enroll in additional educational laser seminars to remain current with treatment protocols and technologic advances.

In addition to the issue of medical staff training, the office staff also require special skills to answer prospective patients' questions concerning the treatment or to field telephone calls appropriately. In other words, it is simply not enough to have a well-trained surgical staff if your office staff is unable to handle the multitude of questions that are commonly asked by patients contemplating an initial consultation and possibly treatment. Thus, receptionists and secretaries who are responsible for making appointments should also know which lesions are treatable by lasers, the approximate number of sessions generally required for treatment, and the general array of lasers that can be used. Of course, they can not and *should not* substitute the information that is provided during a patient consultation, but their knowledge and its delivery can influence a patient's decision to actually schedule an appointment with the physician.

Finally, how the information is delivered is of little help if an appointment cannot be booked because of lack of time in the schedule. A good way to avoid unnecessary waiting lists and the possibility of losing a patient who is anxious to begin treatment is to dedicate at least 1 day a week to the evaluation and treatment of patients who desire laser therapy.

▶ Market Considerations

Just as it is important to determine the capability of your office and staff to handle the addition of laser technology, it is equally important to assess its impact on your local market. For instance, a regional market that is already saturated with numerous laser facilities may not justify the addition of yet another laser, whereas a community without any or with only a limited number of lasers could easily handle the addition of a laser center. On the other hand, a community with few or no lasers that is not technologically sophisticated may not be amenable to the benefits of laser surgery regardless of the relative need.

Competition in the community is one aspect of your market evaluation, but professional competition is another. In the past, for instance, reconstructive plastic surgeons and pediatricians have left the bulk of laser surgery to more specialized dermatologists and cosmetic plastic surgeons. With the advent of newer, less expensive, and less difficult (perceptually) laser technology, however, these same physicians, along with ophthalmologists, dentists, and a host of other practitioners, are now performing these procedures themselves. The perceived ease of laser surgery has pervaded the market from physician to patient, which has no doubt made laser surgery more accessible, but has also increased the risk of complications by insufficiently trained physicians. That is not to say that more physicians cannot perform these procedures. Because there are no board or training requirements, however, it is incumbent on each treating physician to have sufficient training before embarking in this specialty with its inherent risks.

Fortunately, there are instances when competing laser facilities could actually work together. Because some lesions, such as multicolored tattoos, require more than one laser for successful removal, a laser center with only a neodymium yttrium-aluminum-garnet (Nd:YAG) laser may need to refer to another center with either a Q-switched ruby or alexandrite laser to remove any green pigment that cannot be eradicated by the Nd:YAG system. Both patients and physicians benefit from this collaboration.

▶ Financial Considerations

Lasers are expensive to obtain and maintain, so a careful analysis of your financial capabilities is necessary before committing to a purchase or lease arrangement. Most practitioners find that leasing the laser equipment affords them more flexibility with regard to upgrade and trade-in capabilities. In addition, leasing does not require the initial investment of capital, which is especially important for new practitioners. The finance rates offered by most leasing companies are so favorable that the monthly payments are lower than with purchasing. In addition, with leasing, immediate business deductions can be taken, rather than claiming the depreciation of the purchased equipment over its useful life-span. In addition, laser technology advances so rapidly that your laser may be obsolete before you anticipate. Thus, leasing holds several advantages. On the other hand, if you live in a country where the ability to upgrade or obtain adequate leasing arrangements is limited, such as in Europe or Asia, equipment purchase makes the most sense.

The addition of yet a third option, that of renting mobile laser units on a daily basis, could be the best way for a new laser practitioner to assess whether a particular laser is a good investment for the practice and whether it would be beneficial to become more financially involved in an extensive laser program. Most of the mobile laser services provide a group of lasers on a predetermined schedule (e.g, weekly, biweekly, monthly) to an office for a fee that is billed directly to the patient, the doctor, or both. The treating physician also charges a treatment fee to the patient. This arrangement only works when patients are amenable to scheduling their surgeries on predetermined dates. It is not advantageous when patients are unwilling to return on a separate date for the procedure or when a laser is needed in an emergent situation (eg, a rapidly proliferating hemangioma). In most instances, however, mobile laser units allow a physician time to become familiar with the laser technology and to build a laser practice without the financial risk inherent with leasing or buying equipment.

In addition to the lease or purchase payments, other expenses related to the acquisition of lasers include annual service contract fees and the cost of disposable parts or additional equipment. Because lasers are prone to breaking down, it is unwise to disregard the need for an annual service contract. The cost of fixing a laser on a case-by-case basis adds up to a bigger expense than investing in a maintenance contract—similar to fixing a car without insurance. Most service or maintenance contract fees range from $10,000 to $20,000 annually, so this is not a fly-by expense. Other expenses pertaining to the laser equipment include dye cartridges (for the pulsed dye laser systems) and smoke evacuators (for the carbon dioxide laser systems). These extra expenses add up, so they should be given full consideration before making the decision to lease or buy a laser.

Another expense that may be overlooked is malpractice insurance. Liability coverage for laser surgery may increase your regular insurance premiums, so it is best to check with your insurance carrier to determine whether your rates will be affected with the addition of laser technology to your practice.

▶ Laser Considerations

Literally hundreds of lasers are available, and choosing the right laser for your practice can be difficult and time-consuming. In addition to considering cost, you must be fully aware of which patients or lesions you will most often be treating. As mentioned earlier, different lasers treat different lesions (Fig. 1-1 and Table 1-3). If you tend to treat many birthmarks, such as port-wine stains, hemangiomas, and café-au-lait macules, you should consider a pulsed dye laser at 585 or 510 nm. If you are primarily consulted for treatment of telangiectasias and solar lentigines, a wide range of lasers (from pulsed dye to quasi-CW copper vapor, KTP, krypton, and argon-pumped dye lasers) could be beneficial. The quasi-CW lasers tend to be less expensive, but they lack the high degree of vascular or pigment specificity that the pulsed dye lasers have, which is needed for safe treatment of large vascular and pigmented birthmarks. The Q-switched ruby, Nd:YAG, and alexandrite lasers can individually treat blue-black tattoos, but the ruby and alexandrite lasers cannot remove red ink, and the Nd:YAG laser cannot remove green ink without the addition of a second laser. So, if you plan on only treating tattoos, you must seriously consider having access to two laser systems. Fortunately, these same Q-

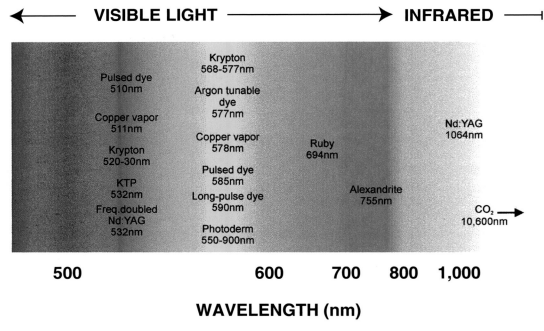

Figure 1-1

Lasers and their wavelengths.

TABLE 1-3. LASER CHECKLIST FOR VARIOUS DERMATOLOGIC LESIONS

Lesion	510-nm Pulsed Dye	511-nm Copper Vapor	520–530-nm Krypton	532-nm Frequency-Doubled ND:YAG	532-nm KTP	568-nm Krypton	577-nm Argon-Pumped Dye	578-nm Copper Vapor	585-nm Pulsed Dye	590–600-nm Long-Pulsed Dye	550–900-nm Photo Derm	694-nm Ruby	755-nm Alexandrite	1064-nm Nd:YAG	10,600-nm Pulsed CO_2	Comments
Vascular																
Facial telangiectasia	✓	✓	✓		✓	✓	✓	✓	✓							
Leg telangiectasia	✓															
Port-wine stain									✓	✓	✓					
Hemangioma							✓		✓	✓	✓					
Poikiloderma							✓		✓	✓	✓					
Pigment																
Solar lentigines		✓	✓		✓							✓	✓	✓		
Café-au-lait		✓		✓												
Nevus of Ota												✓	✓	✓		
Benign nevus				✓								✓	✓	✓		
Melasma																Does not respond to any laser treatment
Tattoos																
Black/blue												✓	✓	✓		
Green												✓	✓			
Red				✓												Tattoo ink darkens after laser irradiation
Fleshtone	✓															
Scars																
Hyperpigmented	✓															
Erythematous									✓							
Hypertrophic									✓							
Keloid									✓							
Atrophic									✓						✓✓	
Hypopigmented																Combination treatment with CO_2 followed by 585 pulsed dye
Others																
Striae									✓							
Rhytides									✓						✓✓	
Verrucae															✓✓	Low fluence is best

switched lasers can be used to treat other lesions as well, such as nevi of Ota, solar lentigines, and other benign pigmented lesions. Hypertrophic or keloid scars and recalcitrant verrucae respond favorably to vascular-specific 585-nm pulsed dye laser irradiation; hence, a single laser system can be used to treat various lesions. Finally, if you are primarily interested in resurfacing photodamaged or acne-scarred skin, then your obvious choice would be a high-energy, pulsed, or scanned CO_2 laser.

Although the idea of a two-in-one laser is appealing, the dual laser technology many times lacks specificity for any particular target. An example of this is the copper vapor laser, which emits light at two different wavelengths: a 511-nm green light to treat pigmented lesions and a 578-nm yellow light to treat vascular lesions. The wavelengths are appropriately matched for these lesions, but the quasi-CW nature of the laser limits its appropriateness in the treatment of large vascular and pigmented lesions, such as port-wine stains and café-au-lait macules, because of the potential development of textural changes or scar formation. Thus, the use of this two-in-one laser is best reserved for such small lesions as telangiectasias and solar lentigines. Another problem with two-in-one lasers arises when two distinctly different technologies are contained in the same laser unit, such as the PLTL laser (Candela Laser Corporation, Wayland, MA). In this system, a 510-nm pulsed dye laser is combined with a 755-nm alexandrite laser. Although the combination of wavelengths is optimal for the treatment of multicolored tattoos (the 510-nm laser can treat the red, yellow, and orange pigments that the 755-nm laser cannot treat), this unit is more susceptible to malfunctions because of the existence of two different technologies (liquid and solid-state delivery systems).

When choosing a laser, in addition to considering the cost and effectiveness of the different laser systems, you should also investigate the longevity and durability of each laser company under consideration. Nothing would be worse than acquiring a laser, only to find out that the laser company is going out of business or cannot keep pace with ongoing technologic advances. The expense of each laser system warrants investigation not unlike what you would undertake when considering the purchase of a new home.

▶ Marketing Your New Laser

Few patients with laser-amenable lesions are ready for laser treatment for a whole host of reasons—from lack of time for healing, to lack of money for payment, to lack of enthusiasm for undergoing a "novel" treatment. This means that you must generate business from your existing patients or within the greater community. Fortunately, there are multiple ways of marketing your new laser facility (Fig. 1-2).

The first and easiest way to market is by word-of-mouth. It is also the least expensive. By simply talking up the attributes of dermatologic laser surgery to patients, friends, and family, you could generate several referrals. Another way to get the word out is through informational letters sent to existing patients and referring physicians. The letter should be personal but also contain valuable information relating to the conditions that can be treated as well as the expected clinical results and the reasons why laser therapy is a superior treatment.

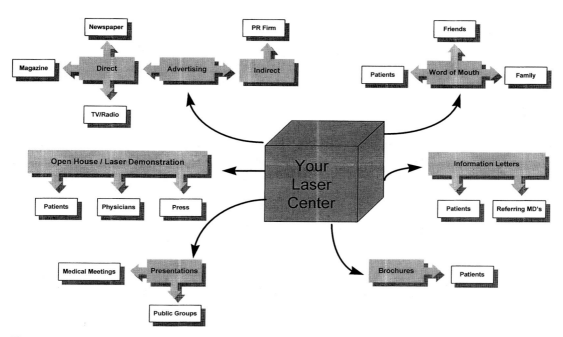

Figure 1-2
Laser marketing strategies.

Promotional brochures and newsletters that outline the new services and contain before-and-after laser treatment photographs are another important marketing tool. These are often supplied by laser manufacturers but can be custom-designed for a more personal presentation. Prominently displaying these items in your waiting room or mailing them to former and new patients may prompt patient interest. Patients are often surprised to learn that there is a treatment that could rid them of such "simple" lesions as solar lentigines and telangiectasias, as well as more complex lesions as tattoos and birthmarks. Without being prompted by a brochure or newsletter, they probably would remain unaware of the full range of treatment options available.

Presentations at local medical society or hospital division meetings can educate your colleagues about the merits of laser surgery and generate additional referrals. Nurses, residents, and fellows in training can be excellent referral sources. Similar lectures at special groups (eg, churches, beauty salons, health clubs) or service clubs (eg, Lion's, Rotary) are another excellent way to educate the public and possibly to gain extra referrals.

"Open houses," whereby you invite other physicians, the public, or press in for a tour of your laser facility and a laser demonstration could lead to referrals, direct patient consultations, or even an article in a local newspaper or magazine. It gives others a chance to meet you and view the laser without making a commitment.

Direct advertising in newspapers and magazines or on television or radio is an expensive undertaking but is another valuable marketing tool. If direct advertising is not your style, indirect advertising through a public relations consultant may be a more palatable method of sparking media attention on your new laser capabilities. Publicists have several media contacts whom they can access to transmit your message in a more "user-friendly" tone or can set the stage for an appropriate interview with the press.

SAMPLE SOLICITATION LETTER TO PHYSICIANS

Dear Colleague:

In a continuing effort to offer the most advanced laser technology in the area, I am pleased to announce my recent acquisition of the new _____ laser system. This laser provides the latest state-of-the-art technology to complement the existing laser services for *(vascular/ pigmented/tattooed/scarred/other lesions)* that are already available to my patients. The primary application of this new laser is the removal of *(vascular lesions, pigmented lesions, tattoos, scars, rhytides, other)* without producing undesirable side effects, such as scarring or pigmentary changes.

The laser treatment is offered on an outpatient basis and does not require general anesthesia. Topical, intralesional, or intravenous anesthesia can be used on an individual basis. *(Single/Multiple)* laser treatments are typically needed to obtain the optimal degree of clinical improvement.

If you have patients in your practice who might benefit from this new service, I would be happy to help them. Please have them call my office to arrange a consultation. I would also welcome you to visit my office to introduce you formally to cutaneous laser surgery and its capabilities.

Sincerely,

Manual of Cutaneous Laser Techniques, by Tina S. Alster.
Lippincott–Raven Publishers, Philadelphia © 1997.

CHAPTER 2

PREOPERATIVE PATIENT CONSIDERATIONS

Preoperative Patient Questionnaire ► *Patient Education*

Patients who are interested in undergoing laser surgery first need to be adequately prepared for the appropriate laser procedure. Because of the hype surrounding cutaneous laser surgery, most patients are ill-prepared for the treatment. Patients often mistakenly think that the laser surgery is "easy in, easy out." In other words, most patients believe that they could have the treatment during their lunch hour and then return to work with narry a trace of the original lesion or any treatment side effect. Unfortunately, most of the lasers do not allow for this amount of postoperative ease. Although most lesions do not require more than 30 minutes to treat, healing of the resultant purpura, crusting, or serous discharge (depending on the laser used) typically takes 1 to 2 weeks. Thus, during a patient's initial consultation, several items pertaining to the laser procedure should be reviewed.

▽

PREOPERATIVE PATIENT CHECKLIST

▶ Complete patient medical history, including current medications and allergies
▶ Full-body dermatologic examination
▶ Preoperative photographs
▶ Patient education
  • Before-and-after treatment photographs of similar lesions
  • Video demonstration of laser procedure
  • Preoperative and postoperative information sheets for appropriate laser
  • Informational brochure
  • Verbal instruction
  • Question-and-answer session
▶ Preoperative skin care recommendations
▶ Informed consent reviewed and signed

△

▶ Preoperative Patient Questionnaire

What is the patient's primary concern? Are the lesions amenable to laser treatment?

It is not always evident at first glance what lesions are the cause of the patient's concern. The severely photodamaged facial skin with prominent solar lentigines and rhytides may have drawn your attention, but the patient may be concerned instead about the linear telangiectasias in the perinasal creases or the scattered angiomas that had been increasing in number and size on the trunk. It is proper, therefore, that you first focus on those areas for which the patient has sought your medical expertise. Even though many dermatologic lesions are now considered to be treated most successfully with lasers (Table 2-1), it is important that all treatment options, including their relative benefits and risks, be discussed with the patient.

Does the patient have other skin lesions that are of medical concern or that could be amenable to laser treatment?

Once the patient's primary concern has been addressed, it is then appropriate to discuss the other cutaneous lesions that could benefit from laser treatment. More importantly, lesions found during the patient's general skin examination that are suggestive of malignancy should be documented and biopsied for histopathologic examination. Keratoses indicating excessive actinic damage should be pointed out to the patient, and an appropriate word of caution regarding their malignant potential should be given.

TABLE 2–1. **INDICATIONS FOR LASER TREATMENT**

Lesion Type	Primary Indications	Secondary Indications
Vascular	Port-wine stains Hemangiomas Facial telangiectasias Cherry angiomas Pyogenic granulomas	Kaposi's sarcoma Leg telangiectasias
Pigmented	Lentigines Cafe-au-lait macules Nevus of Ota or Ito	Nevus spilus Becker's nevus Melanocytic nevi
Tattoos	Professional Amateur Traumatic	Cosmetic
Scars	Hypertrophic Atrophic Erythematous Pigmented	Keloid
Rhytides	Perioral Periorbital	Nasolabial folds Forehead Glabella
Other	Xanthelasma Appendageal tumors	Verrucae Keratoses

Has the patient ever had the lesions treated?

Patients with facial telangiectasias may have had electrosurgery in the past, which could have resulted in fibrosis of the surrounding skin, making it more difficult for vascular-specific lasers to achieve an adequate depth of tissue penetration because of the change in skin optics. Although previous sclerotherapy of leg telangiectasias does not usually lead to fibrosis, it often leads to the development of hyperpigmentation due to hemosiderin deposition, which could also impede the penetration and overall effectiveness of a vascular-specific laser. Similarly, solar lentigines that have been treated with cryotherapy may not only have residual pigment, but also may be hypopigmented and fibrotic in areas that received more aggressive treatment. These areas may be less amenable to pigment-specific laser irradiation. Hypertrophic scars and keloids that have been treated with intralesional cortisone or silicone gel sheeting remain responsive to irradiation with a 585-nm pulsed dye laser; however, atrophic scars that had been previously dermabraded or peeled with phenol may be harder to vaporize because of the resultant fibrosis in the treated skin. Also, hypopigmentation may become unmasked after laser resurfacing of those scars that had received prior dermabrasion or phenol peels.

Does the patient have a history of herpes labialis?

Although cutaneous lasers typically do not emit light in the ultraviolet portion of the electromagnetic spectrum, which is known to reactivate herpes simplex virus (HSV) infections, the trauma from laser treatment alone may cause HSV reactivation. A positive history of herpes labialis is of more concern when CO_2 laser resurfacing is performed because the entire skin is deepithelialized during the procedure, and spread or reactivation of HSV has been known to occur. Prophylactic acyclovir or other antiherpetic is thus prescribed for patients with a positive history of labial HSV who plan to undergo CO_2 laser resurfacing.

Are there any other medical conditions or medications that could affect laser treatment, such as autoimmune disease, immunodeficiency, steroid or isotretinoin (Accutane) use?

Patients with scleroderma, lupus, and especially vitiligo may have an exacerbation of their conditions, especially after CO_2 laser resurfacing, which is much more invasive than procedures performed by other dermatologic lasers. Patients with these conditions, as well as those with immune deficiency, should be cautioned that laser resurfacing could unmask or worsen their diseases or make them an easy target for secondary infection. Nonresurfacing lasers have not been known to cause any of these side effects or complications. The prior use of isotretinoin should also be ascertained so that a proper period of time can pass before laser resurfacing. By delaying laser treatment by a year or more after a course of isotretinoin, the risk of hypertrophic scarring, which is known to occur in these patients after dermabrasion, should no longer be increased.

Does the patient have the correct skin type for laser treatment?

Patients with lighter skin tones (skin phototypes I and II) are the best candidates for most laser treatments because of the decreased risk of pigmentary alteration postoperatively. Patients with darker skin tones can also be treated, but they must be prepared for the higher risk of posttreatment hyperpigmentation (25% to 40%), which can take several months to fade. The fading process can be shortened with the use of hydroquinone-containing creams and application of mild peeling agents.

Does the patient have realistic expectations of the treatment?

Patients who think that only one laser treatment will result in flawless skin are unrealistic in their expectations. Other patients, understandably, find it difficult to believe that so many laser treatments will be required to remove "only a small tattoo" that took a mere 30 minutes to put on. Similarly, some patients expect that small solar lentigines should also be removed without any sequelae and in a single session. Patients need to be made fully aware that most dermatologic lesions require *several* laser sessions to obtain the desired clinical outcome and that each treatment session is accompanied by discomfort, skin discoloration, and prolonged healing time. If, after adequate explanations have been given regarding the anticipated treatment, the patient continues to exhibit unrealistic expectations, then the patient should not be treated.

The best patients for laser treatment can be summarized as follows:

Ideal Candidates
▶ Patients with lesions amenable to laser treatment
▶ Patients with pale skin tones (skin phototypes I, II)
▶ Patients who understand treatment protocol and risks
▶ Patients with realistic expectations of treatment
▶ Patients who will comply with advised postoperative skin care and follow-up

Less-Than-Ideal Candidates
▶ Patients with lesions that are less responsive or show unpredictability to laser treatment
▶ Patients with darker skin tones (skin phototypes III, IV, V)
▶ Patients with limitations in comprehension
▶ Patients who travel long distances for treatment (compliance issues)

▶ Patient Education

Vascular Lesions

The type of vascular lesion (ie, involving large- or small-caliber vessels) as well as its location can determine whether a particular vascular-specific laser is suitable. Small- to medium-caliber vessels that comprise port-wine stains, hemangiomas, and the telangiectasias seen in poikiloderma and rosacea are most amenable to 585-nm pulsed dye laser treatment. A long-pulse laser or photothermal sclerosis using a noncoherent pulsed beam works best for leg telangiectasias, and quasi–continuous wave lasers (ie, copper vapor, KTP, krypton) can treat larger-caliber facial telangiectasias.

Because most vascular lesions require more than one laser treatment and at least 6 weeks between treatments for optimal tissue healing, it is important that patients are fully aware not only of the initial healing time (which averages 7 to 10 days postoperatively), but also of the overall time needed for the entire treatment protocol. In addition to providing this information in written form, it is helpful to review everything verbally while showing typical before-and-after laser treatment photographs of similarly affected patients and viewing the laser procedure on videotape.

Pigmented Lesions

Whether a pigmented lesion is superficial or deep determines which pigment-specific laser system is the most suitable for treatment. As is true with vascular lesions, pigmented lesions typically require more than one laser treatment to resolve. Thus, patients should be prepared for the possibility of several laser sessions, especially if they have a pigmented birthmark, such as a café-au-lait macule or nevus of Ota. An information form outlining these facts, a video demonstration of the laser procedure, and a viewing of representative before-and-after laser treatment photographs are all helpful educational tools.

INFORMATION SHEET: VASCULAR LESIONS

You have a vascular lesion (port-wine stain, hemangioma, telangiectasia, angioma), which is made up of a network of blood vessels. These vessels are close to the skin surface, causing your skin to be colored pink, red, or purple. Several treatments, including surgery and skin grafting, injections (sclerotherapy), electrosurgery, freezing (cryotherapy), and x-rays, have been used to treat these types of lesions in the past, with variable results.

Lasers that produce a beam of yellow light can selectively destroy blood vessels and have been shown to treat vascular lesions effectively. Multiple laser treatments are usually necessary to destroy a vascular lesion completely. Most telangiectasias, or spider veins, may need only one to four laser treatments, whereas port-wine stains require an average of nine to twelve treatments for significant lightening. The power of the laser must be individualized for each patient, and repeated treatments over the same skin area every 6 to 8 weeks may be required. A local anesthetic cream can be used to minimize the rubber band–like snapping sensation of the laser. Young children may require a sedative or intravenous anesthesia. Laser-treated skin usually is severely bruised (or purpuric) for 1 to 2 weeks after laser treatment.

Existing laser research and clinical evidence indicate that laser surgery is safe, but there is no guarantee that laser treatment will treat your condition completely. Although side effects from this procedure are minimal, there is a small risk that the following could occur:

- ► Skin lightening (hypopigmentation)
- ► Skin darkening (hyperpigmentation)
- ► Infection
- ► Skin texture change
- ► Scarring
- ► Swelling
- ► Allergic reaction to ointment
- ► Activation of cold sores
- ► Incomplete removal of lesion

INFORMATION SHEET: PIGMENTED LESIONS

You have a tan, blue-gray, or brown skin mark or lesion that is caused by a deposit of pigmented cells (melanocytes) at various depths under the skin surface. Before the development of pigment-specific lasers, most pigmented skin lesions could only be treated with surgical excision, often leading to scar formation. Certain lasers can now focus a green or red beam of light on the unwanted pigment in your skin and destroy it without damaging your normal skin. The following factors should be considered in your decision to undergo laser treatment:

1. Multiple laser treatments are usually necessary (especially for pigmented birthmarks, such as café-au-lait spots and nevi of Ota, which can require six or more laser treatments).
2. Treatments are usually scheduled at 6- to 8-week intervals.
3. The impact of the laser feels like a snap of a rubber band. Although most people find the sensation mildly uncomfortable without the need for any anesthesia, some patients with larger marks or who are more sensitive may require an anesthetic cream or injection before treatment.
4. Immediately after treatment, there may be swelling, bruising, or crusting and scabbing, which can persist for 1 to 2 weeks.
5. Fading of the treated lesion can continue for up to 6 months after laser treatment in some instances.
6. Although existing laser research and clinical evidence indicate that laser surgery is safe, there is no guarantee that laser treatment will be able to treat your condition completely.
7. Although the side effects of this procedure are minimal, there is a small risk that the following complications could occur:
   - Skin texture change or scarring
   - Dyspigmentation (skin lightening or darkening)
   - Infection
   - Incomplete removal of pigmented lesion
   - Allergic reaction to ointment

Tattoos

Depending on the type of tattoo (professional, amateur, cosmetic, or traumatic) and the colors in the tattoo, one or more tattoo-specific lasers may be needed for treatment. It is important to determine preoperatively what type of tattoo is present, whether it has been treated previously, and if any allergic reaction ever occurred within the tattoo. Some patients already gone to extreme lengths to rid themselves of a tattoo—even attempting to burn them off with a hot knife, cigarette embers, or flaming match. Tissue fibrosis or scar formation would be the typical result of such actions and could lead to attenuation of the proposed laser treatment. Similarly, some patients have had portions of their tattoos surgically removed with partial (or staged) excisions or chemabrasions, which also can result in scar formation within the residual tattoo. Still others have had fleshtone or white pigments injected into the original tattoo in an attempt at camouflage; this could present a problem when laser treatment is initiated because iron- or titanium oxide-containing inks common in cosmetic tattoos can darken after Q-switched laser irradiation. Finally, some patients have had their original tattoos retattooed to mask an unwanted name or design, but instead increased the overall pigment burden in their skin.

As with vascular and pigmented lesions, patients should be forewarned that most, if not all, tattoos require multiple laser sessions for removal and that the sensation experienced with each treatment feels similar to that felt when receiving the tattoo (ie, hot pinpricks or bacon grease hitting the skin). In addition to a verbal explanation, a written information sheet should be provided, and a display of clinical photographs depicting similar tattoos at various stages of laser treatment should be viewed. A video demonstration of the actual laser procedure also helps to prepare patients for the treatment.

Scars

Different types of scars require different laser technologies, so it is imperative to categorize the scar in question correctly. Because hypertrophic and keloid scars tend to recur after traditional excisional or vaporizing treatments, these scars are best treated with a 585-nm pulsed dye system, which does not vaporize or injure the skin surface. Atrophic scars, on the other hand, respond well to CO_2 laser resurfacing (see Rhytides for proper patient information). Patients with hypertrophic and keloid scars have often failed other forms of treatment, such as topical or intralesional steroids and silicone gel treatment, which fortunately do not interfere with subsequent laser treatment, as do many other treatments. Patients should be informed that the laser treatment will feel like a succession of rubber band snaps and that the scar will appear purple or black after treatment for about 1 to 2 weeks. An informational sheet that outlines the procedure, healing time, and risks should be provided as well as a full verbal explanation of events. Representative photographs depicting similar scars at various stages of treatment should be viewed, in addition to an educational video, to maximize the patient's understanding of the procedure before undergoing treatment.

INFORMATION SHEET: TATTOOS

A tattoo is created by depositing various colored pigments under the skin surface for decorative or cosmetic purposes. Sometimes, a tattoo can be caused by an explosion or a fall on asphalt, when pieces of metal, dirt, or carbon become lodged under the skin. Many methods have been tried to remove tattoos, including surgical excision, use of various acids and bleaching agents, destruction by heat or cold, overtattooing with flesh-colored pigment, sanding or dermabrading, and various older laser therapies. Many times, these treatments were ineffective or led to significant scarring. Q-switched lasers represent the latest, state-of-the-art technology specifically designed for tattoo treatment. The following factors should be considered in your decision to undergo this laser treatment:

1. Multiple treatments will be necessary (multicolored professional tattoos typically require eight or more laser treatments, whereas amateur or traumatic blue-black tattoos may need as few as two to six treatments).
2. Treatments are usually scheduled at 6- to 8-week intervals, but this interval can be longer or shorter, depending on your individual response.
3. The sensation produced by each laser impact has been likened to that of hot bacon grease hitting the skin. Some people do not require any anesthesia, while others may desire the use of an anesthetic cream or injection before the procedure.
4. Immediately after treatment, there may be swelling, bruising, or crusting and scabbing, which can persist for 1 to 2 weeks.
5. Significant fading of the tattoo can continue for up to 6 months after laser treatment in some instances.
6. Although existing laser research and clinical evidence indicate that laser surgery is safe, there is no guarantee that laser treatment will be able to eliminate your tattoo completely.
7. Although the side effects of this procedure are minimal, there is a small risk that the following could occur after laser treatment:
   - Skin texture change or scarring
   - Dyspigmentation (skin lightening or darkening)
   - Infection
   - Incomplete removal of tattoo (tattoo shadow remains)
   - Allergic reaction to topical ointment or to shattered tattoo ink particles
   - Darkening of fleshtone, white, rust, or brown tattoo pigments (seen primarily in cosmetic tattoos—eyeliner, lipliner)

INFORMATION SHEET: SCARS

A scar can develop in the skin any time there is injury or trauma to the skin. Sometimes, a more severe type of scar develops, which may be red and raised (*hypertrophic*) or grow into a large nodule that extends beyond the margins of the original wound (*keloid*). Hypertrophic scars and keloids affect an estimated 4.5% to 15% of the population. Treatment methods such as excision, freezing, electrocautery, dermabrasion, and steroid injections have been mostly unsuccessful in the treatment of these scars because of their tendency to recur.

Laser surgery using pulsed laser technology has been shown to improve hypertrophic scars and keloids by reducing their redness and thickness, altering the skin texture to one that is more normal, improving pliability (softness), and eliminating symptoms, such as burning and itching. As few as one or two laser treatments are usually necessary; however, with thicker scars, several more sessions may be needed to achieve the desired amount of scar improvement. The treatments are delivered every 6 to 8 weeks to allow adequate time for proper healing of the skin. Immediately after treatment, the scar appears bruised. The deep purple or black skin color lasts about 1 to 2 weeks, after which time the scar begins to appear less red and becomes flatter and softer. You may notice mild itching during the healing phase, which is a normal response.

Existing laser research and clinical evidence indicate that laser surgery is safe, but there is no guarantee that laser treatment will be able to treat your scars completely. Although the side effects of this procedure are minimal, there is a small risk that complications, such as swelling, infection, and an allergic response to topical ointment, could occur. In patients with darker skin tones, hyperpigmentation (or a brownish skin discoloration) within the laser-treated scar may develop, which will eventually disappear. When used properly, the pulsed laser should not lead to additional scarring.

Rhytides

Patients with rhytides that have been determined to be amenable to laser treatment should receive extensive information about cutaneous laser resurfacing. Because the actual laser procedure is more painful and technically difficult, the involvement of an anesthetist (especially for full-face procedures) may become necessary. Postoperative management is more involved because of the protracted and delicate postoperative course. The importance of ample preoperative patient education cannot be overemphasized. Most helpful is for patients to view a videotape of the procedure, followed by a step-by-step pictorial guide of various postoperative stages of the healing skin. Patients find it comforting to be given the opportunity to speak with others who have already undergone the procedure. As always, written and verbal explanations of the technology, procedure, anesthetic considerations, and expected postoperative course are crucial.

INFORMATION SHEET: LASER RESURFACING

The carbon dioxide (CO_2) laser has been a popular surgeon's tool during the past several years. Its use in cosmetic surgery, however, had been limited because of the risk of scarring and pigmentary skin changes that resulted from the deep thermal damage (or heat buildup) it produced in the skin. New pulsed and scanned CO_2 lasers have eliminated this problem by limiting the thermal impact to the most superficial layers of the skin.

When the skin is treated with a pulsed CO_2 laser, a clean layer-by-layer vaporization of the skin occurs. The undesired skin literally evaporates because of the high water content of the epidermis. Therefore, this laser is best used for superficial skin conditions. Fine lines, wrinkles, and indented or pitted scars from acne, surgery, or trauma can be dramatically improved. The skin in these conditions is resurfaced by the vaporizing action of the laser.

The laser procedure is quick, bloodless, and can be performed with simple local or intravenous anesthesia in the office. Immediately after treatment, the skin turns bright red and becomes swollen, and ice packs and healing ointments are used for the first few days. You will return to the office for cleansing facials during the first week. The initial healing process takes place during the first 1 to 2 weeks after treatment, leaving pink, smoother skin. The pink skin eventually normalizes in color, matching the surrounding skin during the next few months. It is typical for a patient to return to work and social activities with makeup coverage within 1 to 2 weeks after laser treatment.

The risk of complications using this advanced laser technology is minimal, but scarring, skin lightening or darkening, sharp demarcation lines, infection, allergic reaction to a topical or oral medication, and cold sore activation can occur. We will take all necessary precautions to prevent the development of any untoward side effects.

Laser Hair Removal

Patients with unwanted or excessive hair growth have many treatment options, but laser-assisted hair removal may provide them with a longer-lasting reduction or even elimination in hair growth. Previous treatments such as electrolysis should be documented because the fibrosis that may have resulted from previous treatment may attenuate subsequent laser treatment or could be an indication of a particularly recalcitrant hirsute region. In certain regions, such as the chin and upper lip, hair is notoriously difficult to eradicate.

Regardless of the region being treated, patients should be prepared for the possibility that several laser sessions may be necessary to achieve the desired amount of hair removal. After each session, hair regrowth is expected to be slower and thinner. Patients should have the procedure explained to them verbally and pictorially. Written information sheets can also be provided.

INFORMATION SHEET: ANESTHESIA

For your comfort and safety, your laser surgeon has requested that a Certified Registered Nurse Anesthetist be with you during your surgery to administer the necessary medications and monitor your vital signs. The anesthetist will meet with you on the morning of your surgery, review your history, and ask you questions about your medical health to select the appropriate anesthetics for you during your planned laser procedure. You will also have the opportunity to have all your questions regarding the anesthesia answered at that time.

During the procedure, you will receive a local anesthetic with intravenous sedation. This is the most common type of anesthesia used in an outpatient setting and can be related to "twilight" sleep—you will be given a combination of medications that will make you comfortable and generally unaware of what is happening. For example, patients are usually able to respond if spoken to, but will be asleep during the procedure. This is *not* the same as general anesthesia, during which you are completely asleep. Your heart rate, blood pressure, electrocardiogram, oxygenation, and respiration will be closely and continually monitored by the anesthetist.

The anesthetist will remain with you throughout the procedure. After a suitable period of time, depending on your individual response, you will be allowed to leave the office in the company of a responsible adult. You will probably be drowsy and may sleep for several hours after you return home. It is advised that you arrange to have someone with you for the first 24 hours after your surgery to help you to and from the bathroom, prepare your meals, assist with ice packs, and ensure that you take your medications as prescribed. You should not undertake any responsible activity, make any important decisions, exert yourself physically, or drive a motor vehicle for at least 24 hours after your surgery.

You may experience some mild nausea, sore throat, redness or bruising at the intravenous site, and a generalized feeling of being "washed out" for several days. Persistent or severe nausea, vomiting, or bleeding should be reported to the doctor immediately.

You should understand that there is always a slight risk whenever you undergo surgery and that anesthesia and results cannot be guaranteed. If you have any further questions before the anesthetist meets with you, please do not hesitate to call the office.

INFORMATION SHEET: LASER HAIR REMOVAL

Excess hair can be a result of certain hormones, medication use, or genetic predisposition. Of course, even a small amount of hair can be undesirable when it is located in an obvious or unusual area or when it is thick and dark in color.

There are numerous ways to remove unwanted hair, including shaving, waxing, the use of a depilatory cream, and electrolysis. Unfortunately, all of these treatments can only provide temporary results. Even electrolysis has failed to produce permanent hair removal in most cases.

Specific lasers to target hair follicles have been developed to treat unwanted hair effectively.

The following factors should be considered in your decision to undergo this laser treatment:

1. More than one laser treatment should be expected, and many treatment sessions may be required to obtain the amount of hair thinning or elimination that you desire.
2. Treatments can be delivered at any time that hair regrowth is noted. (You do not have to wait a minimum period of time before having another treatment.)
3. The sensation produced by the laser has been likened to that of a sparkler tingling the skin. Certain skin areas may be particularly sensitive (such as the upper lip and bikini area), and you may desire the use of a topical anesthetic cream.
4. Immediately after treatment, there is usually no skin reaction. Sometimes, a patient may experience mild redness and swelling, which typically resolves within a couple of hours.
5. Hair regrowth may occur more quickly in areas known to produce hair rapidly, such as the chin and cheeks, than in regions typically associated with slower hair growth, such as the chest and back. Patients usually report that the hair regrowth is slower, finer in texture, and more sparse after laser treatment.
6. Although existing laser research indicates that laser treatment is a safe and effective method to remove hair, there is no guarantee that laser treatment will be able to eliminate your unwanted hair completely.
7. Side effects of this treatment are minimal and include the following:
   - Incomplete removal of hair
   - Infection
   - Pigment changes (white or dark spots)
   - Folliculitis (from ingrown hairs)
   - Skin burn (from hot wax if waxing is performed concomitantly)
   - Allergy to topical solution or cream

Manual of Cutaneous Laser Techniques, by Tina S. Alster.
Lippincott–Raven Publishers, Philadelphia © 1997.

CHAPTER **3**

LASER TREATMENT OF VASCULAR LESIONS

Lesion Categorization ► *Laser Treatment Options* ►
Preoperative Patient Evaluation ►
Laser Treatment Protocol ► *Treatment Parameters*

The first laser that was developed using the principles of selective photothermolysis was a vascular-specific pulsed dye system. The theory, proposed by Anderson and Parrish in the early 1980s, predicted that chromophores (or targets) in the skin, such as hemoglobin and melanin, could be selectively destroyed by lasers that emit light at particular wavelengths and pulse durations. The localized absorption of laser light energy with subsequent production of heat in the target would cause selective damage without destruction of the normal surrounding and overlying skin. Since the development of the pulsed dye laser, several other lasers have been introduced or reintroduced into the market that also show vascular specificity (Table 3-1).

Although each of these lasers has its advantages (eg, lower cost, less cumbersome, greater reliability, dual wavelength capabilities), no laser has been developed that is any more vascular specific or clinically effective than the pulsed dye laser. Modifications have been made to the original model to make it even more clinically effective and technologically advanced. For instance, the original pulsed dye lasers used a 577-nm wavelength (corresponding to the third absorption peak of oxyhemoglobin) and a 5-mm spot size and operated at a rate of 1 pulse every 3 seconds. The current model uses a 585-nm wavelength (allowing for slightly deeper absorption without loss of vascular specificity), a 10-mm spot size (also permitting deeper dermal penetration and fewer pulses required to treat a specific area), and a 1 pulse per second (1 Hz) delivery rate (allowing for quicker treatment sessions). Continued modifications of this pulsed dye system, as well as the development

TABLE 3-1. **VASCULAR-SPECIFIC LASERS**

Laser Type	Laser Specifics	Advantages	Disadvantages
Frequency-doubled Nd:YAG	532 nm; Q-switched	No purpura; good for large vessels	Less vascular-specific; not good for children with large lesions (eg, port-wine stain)
KTP	532 nm; quasi-CW	No purpura; good for large vessels	Less vascular-specific; not good for children with large lesions (eg, port-wine stain)
Krypton	568 nm; quasi-CW	Dual wavelength (520–530 nm); no purpura; good for large vessels	Less vascular-specific; not good for children with large lesions (eg, port-wine stain)
Argon-pumped tunable dye	577 nm; quasi-CW	No purpura; good for large vessels	Less vascular-specific; not good for children with large lesions (eg, port-wine stain)
Copper vapor	578 nm; quasi-CW	No purpura; good for large vessels; dual wavelength (511 nm)	Less vascular-specific; not good for children with large lesions (eg, port-wine stain)
Flashlamp-pumped pulsed dye	585 nm; pulsed	Best vascular specificity; safe in children	Produces purpura
Long-pulsed dye	590 nm; pulsed	Good vascular specificity; deeper penetration	Limited clinical studies; produces mild purpura
Photoderm	550–900 nm; pulsed	No purpura; deeper penetration	Not well understood; treatment parameters need refinement

of other lasers with longer pulses and elliptical handpieces, may produce an even better vascular lesion treatment option in the near future. Before determining which laser would be most beneficial for a particular vascular lesion, however, it is best to determine the proper categorization of the lesion.

▶ Lesion Categorization

Vascular lesions can be grouped according their mode of onset—congenital or acquired:

Congenital
- ▶ Hemangiomas
- ▶ Port-wine stains
- ▶ Venous malformations
- ▶ Lymphangiomas

Acquired
- ▶ Telangiectasias
- ▶ Cherry angiomas
- ▶ Pyogenic granulomas
- ▶ Venous lakes
- ▶ Poikiloderma
- ▶ Kaposi's sarcoma

Congenital lesions, such as hemangiomas and port-wine stains, typically appear on the head and neck and, by definition, are initially seen in infants. Acquired lesions, on the other hand, can arise at any time in a person's life and may be a result of trauma, hormones, actinic skin damage, or syndrome association or may simply be a spontaneous disorder.

Mulliken was the first to propose a classification of vascular lesions based on endothelial cell characteristics. Before this classification scheme, a multitude of confusing and often conflicting and inconsistent terms were used to describe vascular lesions. For example, port-wine stains have been referred to as salmon patches, strawberries, cherry angiomas, and hemangiomas. Mulliken's classification has three major categories of lesions: (1) *hemangiomas*, which show endothelial hyperplasia; (2) *malformations*, which demonstrate normal endothelial cell turnover; and (3) *ectasias*, which show normal endothelial turnover, but also vascular dilation.

Hemangiomas that appear as bright red or bluish nodules typically experience a rapid proliferative phase, growing to an unpredictable size over a variable period of time (Table 3-2). This is followed by a slow involution phase, during which the lesion shrinks over several years, eventually becoming barely perceptible in most cases. Hemangiomas are present at birth in only 30% of cases, but more than 90% arise within the first month of life. They are common benign tumors, seen in 10% of 1-year-old infants. When they are located on the face and are actively growing, they can obstruct normal development by obscuring vision or by impinging on a vital structure, such as the trachea. Other complications, such as ulceration, bleeding, and infection, result when the hemangioma is actively growing and the overlying skin is stretched and fragile.

In contrast, malformations (such as port-wine stains) are always present at birth and are seen in 0.3% to 0.5% of the general population. Unlike hemangiomas, they do not exhibit a proliferative phase, but grow commensurately with the affected patient. Unfortunately, malformations never spontaneously involute. Although they are not associated with obstructive complications, they can lead to

TABLE 3-2. **FEATURES OF CONGENITAL VASCULAR LESIONS**

Feature	Hemangiomas	Port-Wine Stains
Present at birth	30%	100%
Incidence at 1 year	10%–12%	0.3%–0.5%
Female:male ratio	3:1	1:1
Endothelial cell turnover	Increased	Normal
Lesional behavior	Rapid growth phase; spontaneous involution	Grow with individual; never involutes
Head or neck location	60%	85%–90%
Inheritance pattern	None	Multifactorial
Complications	Ulceration, infection, bleeding, visual axis disturbance, congestive heart failure	Glaucoma, seizures, tissue or bone hypertrophy
Associated syndromes	Kasabach-Merritt	Sturge-Weber, Cobb, Klippel-Trenaunay

Modified from Alster TS, Tan OT. Laser treatment of benign cutaneous vascular lesions. Am Fam Phys 44: 547–54, 1991.

underlying soft tissue or bony hypertrophy, nodular development, and color darkening as a result of progressive blood vessel ectasia with advancing age. Like hemangiomas, port-wine stains have not been reported to have a familial predisposition for development; however, detailed family histories obtained from 186 of my patients with port-wine stains have revealed a 20% incidence of familial predisposition. This unusually high incidence is consistent with that of a multifactorial inheritance pattern without evidence of autosomal dominant, recessive, or sex-linked features.

The last category proposed by Mulliken's classification, ectasia, is demonstrated by such lesions as telangiectasias, which are acquired vascular lesions. Telangiectasias can occur singly or as a response to photodamage (as seen in poikiloderma) or as part of a syndrome (eg, Osler-Weber-Rendu) or manifestation of disease (eg, scleroderma, lupus). Most telangiectasias have a tendency to become larger, darker, and more numerous with advancing age because of progressive vessel ectasia.

▶ Laser Treatment Options

As stated earlier, a multitude of vascular lasers are available. Several factors can influence your ultimate decision, including the laser price, its maintenance requirements and reliability, its ability to treat different lesions, and most important, its safety and effectiveness in treating vascular lesions without adverse effects related to the technology.

Although any one of the vascular laser options cited can treat facial telangiectasias well, only the pulsed dye laser can safely and adequately treat port-wine stains in children without significant textural change or scar formation (Table 3-3). Based on the age of the patient and the type of lesion (acquired or congenital), the relative advantages of using one laser system over another becomes readily apparent. Using a particular laser simply because it is more economical or because it does not produce postoperative purpura will be of little consolation to the person

TABLE 3-3. **RESPONSES OF VASCULAR LESIONS TO LASER TREATMENT***

Laser Type	Hemangioma	Port-Wine Stain	Facial Telangiectasia	Leg Telangiectasia	Poikiloderma
Frequency-doubled Nd:YAG	Poor	Poor	Good	Unknown	Unknown
KTP	Fair	Poor	Good	Unknown	Unknown
Krypton	Unknown	Fair	Good	Unknown	Unknown
Argon tunable dye	Fair	Fair	Good	Poor	Unknown
Copper vapor	Fair	Fair	Good	Unknown	Unknown
Flashlamp-pulsed dye	Excellent	Excellent	Excellent	Fair	Excellent
Long-pulsed dye	Good	Good	Excellent	Good	Good
Photoderm	Unknown	Fair	Good	Good	Unknown

* The continuous wave Nd:YAG (1064 nm) and argon (577 nm) lasers have been used in the past to treat hemangiomas with resultant eschar development and undesirable textural changes and scar formation. Despite their ability to "shrink" hemangiomas, they are not currently used in the treatment of these lesions owing to their side effects.

in whom you have produced a scar or significant textural skin change. Any patient would rather deal with the week-long inconvenience of laser-induced purpura than suffer a scar.

Quasi–Continuous Wave Lasers

A variety of quasi–continuous wave (CW) lasers (eg, krypton, KTP, argon-pumped tunable dye, copper vapor) are used to treat facial telangiectasias. Their wavelengths vary from 532 to 578 nm. The longer wavelength lasers, emitting yellow light at 577 to 578 nm, can penetrate the skin more deeply and show greater vascular selectivity than melanin selectivity. The shorter, 532-nm green wavelength tends to be more melanin specific. Quasi-CW lasers are excellent for the treatment of large-caliber telangiectasias primarily because of their ability to produce more heat in deeper vessels. On the other hand, small-caliber telangiectasias or small to medium vessels contained in port-wine stains are better treated with the pulsed dye systems because of improved vascular specificity with limited heat conduction to the surrounding skin.

The quasi-CW lasers are pulsed using a shuttering mechanism, which can produce individual 30-millisecond pulses (argon-pumped tunable dye laser) or trains of 30- to 50-nanosecond pulses at rates of 6000 to 15,000 repetitions per second (copper vapor laser). The rapid delivery of pulses in the copper vapor laser system effectively acts like a CW laser, whereas the 30-millisecond pulse of the argon-pumped tunable dye laser is a thousand times longer in duration than the pulsed dye systems that emit light in 1-microsecond pulses. To comply with the basic principles of selective photothermolysis, both the correct wavelength (to match the target's maximum absorption spectrum) and pulse duration (not to exceed the target's thermal relaxation time) should be chosen. Thus, a quasi-CW laser system can be used to treat large-caliber blood vessels because of the longer thermal relaxation time of the larger target. Smaller-caliber telangiectasias and vessels comprising port-wine stains, however, require much shorter pulse durations for prevention of excessive heat conduction to normal surrounding collagen, which could result in a scar.

Pulsed Lasers

The prototypic pulsed laser is the flashlamp-pumped pulsed dye laser, which was specifically developed for the treatment of cutaneous vascular lesions. The initial model's wavelength, set to 577 nm, corresponded to the third absorption peak of oxyhemoglobin. The wavelength has subsequently been adjusted to 585 nm, which provides for greater depth of dermal penetration without loss of vascular specificity. The pulse duration of 450 microseconds is well within the allowable limit because the thermal relaxation time of small to medium-sized blood vessels ranges 1 to 5 milliseconds. Thus, the heat produced by each laser pulse is confined to the targeted blood vessels and is dissipated before it can diffuse to adjacent normal structures. This vascular selectivity has been confirmed histologically with the immediate appearance of agglutinated red blood cells within the irradiated vessels situated in the papillary and upper reticular dermis. The dermal–epidermal junction remains intact, as does the overlying and surrounding collagen. The damaged blood vessels are replaced with normal dermal structures and capillaries within 1 month after treatment.

Long-pulsed lasers, emitting light at 590 to 600 nm with 1- to 10-millisecond pulses, are used to treat larger-caliber and deep dermal blood vessels. They are also helpful in the treatment of recalcitrant port-wine stains. These port-wine stains have shown a relative unresponsiveness to continued 585-nm pulsed dye laser irradiation, which may be due to the presence of residual deep dermal vessels or thickened vessel walls resulting from previous repetitive laser sessions. Another area in which long-pulsed lasers have shown promise is in the treatment of leg telangiectasias, which are generally of larger caliber with thicker vessel walls.

The Photoderm VL, a noncoherent intense pulsed light source, has also been shown to improve lower extremity telangiectasias and recalcitrant port-wine stains. This laser uses a 550-nm cutoff filter that permits light to be emitted at 550 to 900 nm. The emission of longer wavelengths permits deeper tissue penetration, which probably accounts for the device's effectiveness in these conditions.

▶ Preoperative Patient Evaluation

Patients present for treatment with the smallest telangiectasia to the most disfiguring nodular port-wine stain. It is up to you to determine if they are suitable candidates for laser treatment and whether you have the available technology and skill to treat them.

Several factors are important to consider before discussing a particular patient's treatment options (see Chap. 2). For the treatment of vascular lesions, the following issues should be addressed.

Does the patient have a lesion amenable to vascular-specific laser treatment?

Certainly, a patient with a port-wine stain does not have another viable treatment option without risking excessive scarring or pigmentary alteration. Hemangiomas have been shown to respond favorably to laser treatment, but they often resolve spontaneously by the time a child reaches 9 years of age. Other treatments, such as intralesional or systemic steroid therapy, radiation treatment, and interferon administration, can effect a positive response in these lesions, although there are some significant drawbacks and limitations to these treatments. In these cases, an explanation of all the available treatment options and their advantages and disadvantages is provided. It is less risky to undergo laser treatment than to receive some of these other treatments. I have found that a combination treatment protocol consisting of oral corticosteroids, 1 to 3 mg/kg/day in a single daily dose, and concomitant monthly laser treatments is the most effective management of rapidly proliferating or mixed (superficial and deep) hemangiomas.

Facial telangiectasias, although most selectively treated with a vascular laser, have been eradicated for years with electrodesiccation, but with a higher risk of textural changes. Nonetheless, patients should be aware of this treatment option as well as that of sclerotherapy. Lower-extremity telangiectasias that measure larger than 1 mm in diameter respond best to sclerotherapy. Smaller-caliber or mat telangiectasias, for which sclerotherapy is suboptimal, are good candidates for laser treatment. Poikiloderma is best treated with a vascular-specific laser when most of the lesion has been determined to be vascular rather than pigmented (test for skin blanching on finger compression).

Has the patient received previous treatment to the lesion?

Telangiectasias that have been treated with electrodesiccation can be more difficult to treat with laser therapy because of the development of surrounding tissue fibrosis induced by the previous treatment. Port-wine stains that have been treated with older laser technology, such as CW argon or carbon dioxide lasers, or even less vascular-specific lasers, such as copper vapor or KTP lasers, may have developed mild to severe fibrosis with hypertrophic scarring within the treated areas. Similarly, hemangiomas that have been irradiated or injected with corticosteroids or sclerosants may exhibit variable degrees of fibrosis, requiring adjustments in the energy density chosen for treatment. Previous injection of fleshtone tattoo pigment in an attempt to camouflage a port-wine stain also attenuates subsequent laser treatment.

Has the patient suffered any complications or side effects as a result of the lesion's presence?

Hemangiomas that are actively proliferating can ulcerate and develop secondary infections. They can also block or impair vital structures, such as the eye and trachea, leading to visual axis disturbances or breathing difficulties. Port-wine stains can develop pyogenic granulomas, which are prone to easy bleeding; they can also develop evidence of soft tissue and bony hypertrophy, producing further asymmetry. Cherry angiomas in areas prone to trauma or repeated irritation can lead to bleeding. The psychological impact of a vascular birthmark is beyond the scope of this book, but it should not be underestimated or ignored. A child with a disfiguring birthmark always elicits sympathy, but the impact that a birthmark has had on an adult who has already suffered a lifetime of discrimination and ridicule should also be given full consideration.

What is the patient's skin type?

Vascular lesions in patients with darker skin tones can be treated, but more care is taken in selecting an appropriate energy and in determining proper treatment intervals, for two reasons. First, because the overlying melanin (of which there is more in darker skin tones) is a competing chromophore for the yellow laser light, it may shield the underlying vascular lesion and reduce the amount of effective light reaching the lesion. Second, patients with darker skin tones have a greater likelihood of postoperative hyperpigmentation or hypopigmentation. Because all treatment-induced pigmentary alterations should be completely resolved before the delivery of additional laser treatment to effect the optimal result from each session, longer intervals may be necessary between laser treatments.

Does the patient have realistic expectations of the laser treatment?

Patients with telangiectasias should be prepared for one to three laser treatments, but those with port-wine stains and hemangiomas typically require six or more treatments for significant clinical clearing. Those patients with port-wine stains located in certain areas (such as the medial cheeks, upper lip, or distal extremities) should be prepared for additional treatments. Although it is customary to tell patients that the younger one is, the better the port-wine stain response to laser treatment, my experience with more than 300 port-wine stain patients has not substantiated this rhetoric. Most adult port-wine stain patients have stable lesions during the 1- to 2-year treatment protocol, thereby permitting efficient elimination of lesional vessels. The progressive ectasia observed in children's port-wine stains between laser treatments, on the other hand, may be responsible for the slower response rates observed in some children.

In general, patients with congenital lesions are usually so excited by the prospect of having their birthmarks removed that they may fail to appreciate the fact that multiple treatments are necessary. They may show extreme disappointment when only a fraction of their original lesion is removed after the first treatment session, even if it is significant. Thus, proper patient preparation and expectation remain paramount to a treatment's success.

I have found the use of a checklist to be helpful when first evaluating a patient for vascular laser treatment. The checklist remains part of the patient's medical record and can be referred to or updated during subsequent patient visits.

Once a patient has been determined to be an appropriate candidate for vascular laser treatment, detailed pretreatment education is initiated. Information sheets are provided and reviewed with the patient (see Chap. 2), and preoperative photographs are obtained. Taking photographs at each office visit provides a chronologic pictorial of the patient's response to laser treatments. It can be difficult for patients to continue with the treatments when they do not notice their day-by-day improvement. Thus, showing them what the lesion looked like at their previous visits gives them impetus to continue with their proposed treatment course. Computer and video technology that captures and stores clinical photographs is widely available (eg, Mirror Image). The clinical images are instantly available (thereby eliminating the need for film processing), and patients can view their before-and-after photographs or a series of clinical images side by side. Computer printouts of the images can be generated that are similar in quality to laboratory-processed color photographs.

Before beginning laser treatment, the patient must sign an informed consent and be given the opportunity to ask further questions. Only then can laser treatment proceed.

LASER TREATMENT OF VASCULAR LESIONS: PREOPERATIVE CHECKLIST

Type of vascular lesion:

_____ hemangioma	_____ Kaposi's sarcoma
_____ port-wine stain	_____ telangiectasia
_____ angioma	_____ spider veins (legs)
_____ venous lake	_____ pyogenic granuloma
_____ poikiloderma	_____ other (_____)

Location of lesion:

_____ scalp	_____ arms	_____ back
_____ face	_____ legs	_____ abdomen
_____ neck	_____ hands	_____ buttocks
_____ chest	_____ feet	_____ other (_____)

Prior treatments (list with dates): _____

Any history of:

_____ seizures	_____ glaucoma	_____ mental retardation
_____ herpes labialis	_____ ulceration	_____ lesional bleeding

Medical problems (list): _____

Allergies: _____

Current medications: _____

Information sheet given to patient and thoroughly reviewed _____ (initials/date)

Informed consent reviewed and signed _____ (initials/date)

Preoperative photographs obtained _____ (initials/date)

Laser treatment scheduled:

   Type _____   Date _____

Postoperative skin care reviewed and written instructions given to
   patient _____ (initials/date)

LASER TREATMENT OF VASCULAR LESIONS: INFORMED CONSENT

I, _____, understand that I have a benign vascular lesion called a _____. Dr. _____ has explained to me that although laser surgery is effective in most cases, no guarantees can be made that I will benefit from treatment. I understand that several treatment sessions may be needed to obtain the desired level of improvement. Sometimes, a lesion will not completely clear, but it should appear lighter. Rarely, a vascular lesion may not respond to laser treatment at all.

The commonest side effects and complications of this laser treatment are:

1. *Pain.* The snapping and burning sensation of each laser pulse may produce a minimal to moderate amount of discomfort. An anesthetic cream or injection may be used to block the pain if desired.
2. *Bruising.* Immediately after the laser treatment, the area will appear gray or blue-black in color. The discoloration will fade during the next 7 to 10 days.
3. *Swelling.* Areas most likely to swell are under the eyes and neck. The swelling subsides within 3 to 5 days with regular ice application.
4. *Blisters or scabs.* These rarely develop and can take 1 to 2 weeks to resolve.
5. *Skin darkening (hyperpigmentation).* This can occur in the treated areas and fades within 2 to 6 months. This reaction is more common in patients with olive or dark skin tones and can worsen if the laser-treated area is exposed to the sun.
6. *Skin lightening (hypopigmentation).* This can occur in an area of skin that has already received several treatments. The light spots usually darken or repigment in 3 to 6 months, but they can be permanent in rare cases.
7. *Scarring.* This is extremely rare after vascular-specific laser therapy but can occur on disruption of the skin's surface. Following all advised postoperative instructions will reduce the possibility of this occurrence.
8. *Lesion persistence.* Some vascular lesions may not go away completely despite the best efforts made by the doctor.

I further understand that, if left untreated, my vascular lesion would not be expected to go away on its own. It also would not pose a medical threat, but it could become darker, larger, or more raised with time.

By providing my signature below, I acknowledge that I have read and understood all of the information written above and feel that I have been adequately informed of my alternative treatment options, the risks of the proposed laser surgery, and the risks of not treating my condition. I hereby freely consent to the laser surgery to be performed by Dr. _____ and authorize the taking of clinical photographs, which will be used solely for my medical records unless my physician deems that their anonymous use (in lectures or scientific publications) could benefit medical research and education. They will not be used for advertising without my written permission.

_____   _____   _____   _____
Patient's or Guardian's Signature   Date   Witness' Signature   Date

► Laser Treatment Protocol

A checklist used at the time of the actual procedure and a treatment log designed for each patient ensures that nothing is mistakenly overlooked and that all laser specifics are properly documented. It is also helpful to dictate an operative report for each procedure, which remains on file in case an insurance company requests one for reimbursement purposes.

LASER TREATMENT OF VASCULAR LESIONS: OPERATIVE CHECKLIST

- ► Vascular laser in "ready" mode, calibrated to correct energy with proper handpiece
- ► Anesthetic cream or makeup completely removed with mild soap and water
- ► Safety goggles or glasses on operating personnel and patient
- ► No flammable substances in operating area
- ► Hair protected with wet gauze or headband
- ► Tissues and ice water available for patient comfort
- ► Hand-held fan to cool patient during treatment
- ► Laser tray: bacitracin, polysporin, or mupirocin (Bactroban) ointment, wet gauze, ice pack, Telfa pad, Vigilon, or other wound dressing, cotton swabs
- ► Written postoperative instructions given to patient
- ► Return appointment scheduled

► Treatment Parameters

Different laser systems are used at different energies, pulse widths, and spot sizes to treat the same vascular lesions. The following sections provide suggested parameters for each laser system. These are *not* fool-proof. Nothing surpasses individualized protocols based on a patient's clinical examination, skin type, history, and tissue response.

LASER TREATMENT OF VASCULAR LESIONS: TREATMENT LOG

Patient name: _____ Age: _____

Skin type: _____

Diagnosis:_____

_____

Previous treatment(s): _____

Treatment #_____ Photos taken: yes/no

Date: _____

    Laser used: _____

    Fluence or power: _____ (J/cm^2 or watts)

    Spot size: _____

    Anesthesia: _____

    Tissue cooling: yes/no

    Location treated: _____

    Area (in cm) treated: _____

    Number of laser pulses: _____

    Total treatment time: _____

    Skin appearance S/P rx: _____

    Complications: _____

    Bacitracin and Telfa pad applied: yes/no

    Return appointment scheduled: _____ (date)

    Home care: Bacitracin/Telfa pad/Vigilon/acetaminophen (circle)

LASER TREATMENT OF VASCULAR LESIONS: SAMPLE OPERATIVE REPORT

Patient name: _____

Diagnosis: _____

Date of operation: _____

Surgeon: _____

Procedure performed: Treatment of _____[lesion] of

the _____ [location] with the _____

laser

Anesthesia: _____

Total anesthesia time: _____

Laser Procedure

The patient was brought into the operating room and placed in a supine
position. Protective goggles were placed on the patient, and hair-bearing areas
were protected. The _____ laser was calibrated
to _____ [energy], and the _____
[lesion] of the _____ [location] (total area
of _____ cm) was treated with a _____-mm spot size. The laser-
irradiated area(s) showed the expected (purpuric/hyperemic/other) tissue
response. The patient tolerated the procedure well.

Total operative time: _____

Postoperative wound dressings: Bacitracin ointment and Telfa pad

Postoperative medications: Acetaminophen, _____ mg orally every 4 to
6 hours as needed

Postoperative disposition of patient: Stable and ambulatory

Follow-up appointment scheduled: 6 to 8 weeks

_____

Surgeon's signature   Date

TABLE 3-4. **LASER TREATMENT OF VASCULAR LESIONS**

Vascular Lesion	Number of Treatments Required
Port-wine stain	6–18 (average, 8–10)
Hemangioma	2–10 (average, 4–6)
Facial telangiectasia	1–3
Leg telangiectasia	1–3
Pyogenic granuloma	1–4
Cherry angioma	1–2
Venous lake	1–4
Kaposi's sarcoma	2–6
Poikiloderma	2–4

Pulsed Lasers

Flashlamp-Pumped Pulsed Dye Laser (585 nm)

Small facial telangiectasias can be treated using a 2-, 3-, 5-, 7-, or 10-mm spot size at fluences ranging from 4 J/cm^2 (with a 10-mm spot) to 8 J/cm^2 (with a 2-mm spot). Typically, only one to three laser treatments are necessary (Table 3-4).

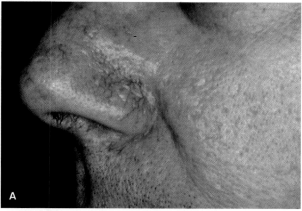

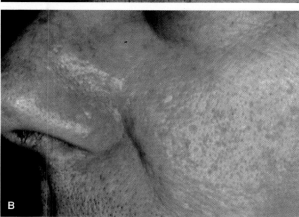

Figure 3-1

A 42-year-old man with perinasal telangiectasias before (*A*) and 4 weeks after (*B*) second 585-nm pulsed dye laser treatment at average fluence 6.75 J/cm^2 using a 7-mm spot. (The quasi-CW lasers—krypton, KTP, copper vapor, or argon tunable dye—can successfully treat these telangiectasias as well.)

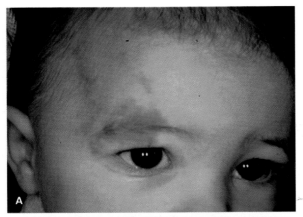

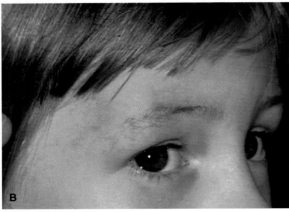

Figure 3-2

Port-wine stain on the brow of a 3-year-old girl before (A) and 6 weeks after (B) fourth 585-nm pulsed dye laser treatment at average fluence 6.5 J/cm^2 using a 5-mm spot size.

Large-caliber telangiectasias are best treated using the largest spot sizes available (7 and 10 mm) to obtain deeper dermal penetration. Similarly, higher fluences (4.5 to 5 J/cm^2 with a 10-mm spot, and 6.5 to 7 J/cm^2 with a 7-mm spot) can effect a purpuric response in the large vessels (Fig. 3-1).

Port-wine stains and hemangiomas are usually treated using a 7- or 10-mm spot size so that fewer laser pulses (or snaps) per session are required and deeper vessels are affected. Initial average energy densities range 4 to 4.75 J/cm^2 with a 10-mm spot and 6 to 7 J/cm^2 with a 7-mm spot (Figs. 3-2 to 3-5). Port-wine stains typically require 8 to 10 laser treatments at 6- to 8-week intervals, whereas hemangiomas require an average of four to six treatments at monthly intervals. Patients with rapidly proliferating or mixed hemangiomas that do not respond to laser treatment alone should be placed on oral corticosteroids, 1 to 3 mg/kg/day in a single dose, until growth is stabilized. The dosage is then tapered every 2 weeks as determined by lesional response.

Although not vascular lesions per se, verrucae that have been recalcitrant to treatment or have recurred after treatment (especially those located in the periungual and plantar regions) are also amenable to 585-nm pulsed dye laser irradiation. They are treated at the highest fluences available—5 J/cm^2 using a 10-mm spot size or 8 J/cm^2 using a 7-mm spot size. Their favorable response to vascular-

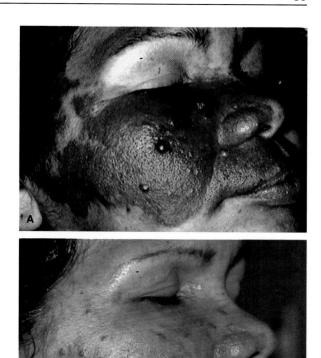

Figure 3-3

A 50-year-old woman with an advanced port-wine stain and pyogenic granulomas before (A) and after (B) eight treatments with the 585-nm pulsed dye laser at average fluence of 6.75 J/cm² using a 7-mm spot.

specific laser treatment is thought to be due to a disruption of the papillary blood supply "feeding" the verrucae, with resultant epidermal necrosis.

Pulsed dye laser spots are placed adjacent to one another in a nonoverlapping fashion to minimize undesirable side effects. Overlapping laser spots, or double-pulsing, causes nonselective tissue heating, which can lead to possible pigmentary or textural changes, such as scarring. An immediate purpuric tissue response should result after 585-nm laser irradiation with a variable degree of reactive hyperemia in the surrounding skin. Delicate or thin tissue areas, such as the infraorbital region, the lips, and neck, may have associated edema. The fragile nature of the anterior chest, neck, and periorbital regions, in particular, require that treatment fluences be decreased by 10% to 20% in these areas. Thus, poikiloderma should be treated with low fluences of 3.75 to 4 J/cm² when using a 10-mm spot, or 4.5 to 5 J/cm² with a 7-mm spot (Fig. 3-6). Surprisingly, because of mucosal optics, the lips do *not* require a reduction in treatment fluences. Thus, venous lakes on the lips can be treated with fluences of 4.5 to 5 J/cm² using a 10-mm spot, or 6.5 to 7.5 J/cm² with a 7-mm spot.

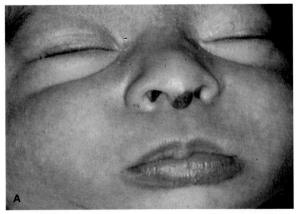

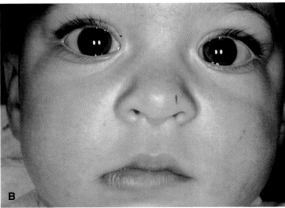

Figure 3-4

A 10-month-old infant with a superficial hemangioma on the nose before (*A*) and 2 months after (*B*) third treatment with the 585-nm pulsed dye laser at average fluence of 6.5 J/cm^2 with a 7-mm spot size.

Long-Pulsed Laser (590 to 600 nm)

Experience with the long-pulsed laser system has been primarily limited to the treatment of leg telangiectasias measuring 0.2 to 1 mm in diameter, which can be effectively cleared within one to three treatments at fluences of 15 to 20 J/cm^2. The longer 1.5-millisecond pulse permits deeper vessel penetration. The use of an elliptical 2×7-mm spot permits selective vessel tracing without production of excessive purpura (Fig. 3-7). Resistant or recalcitrant port-wine stains also show encouraging results using the longer 1.5-millisecond pulse with a 7- or 10-mm spot size.

Photoderm VL (550 to 900 nm)

The Photoderm VL is a pulsed noncoherent light source capable of emitting high fluences at variable pulse durations, intervals, and wavelengths. The rectangular spot size of 8×35 mm used in this device permits the rapid treatment of larger, widespread vessels ranging from 0.1 to 3 mm in diameter. Leg telangiectasias are typically treated using a 550-nm cutoff filter for superficial vessels and a 590-nm cutoff filter for deeper and larger vessels. A regimen that has been shown to achieve

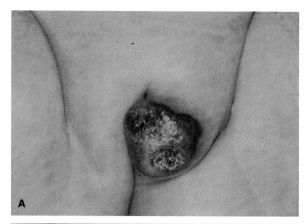

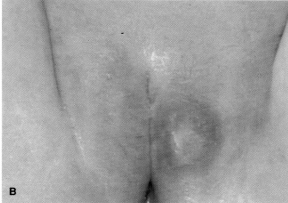

Figure 3-5

A 1-year-old infant with a mixed hemangioma with ulcerations on the vulva before (*A*) and 1 month after (*B*) sixth treatment with the 585-nm pulsed dye laser at average fluence 4 J/cm^2 with a 10-mm spot size.

the best clinical results within two to three treatments separated by 4-week intervals involves using a triple pulse at 20- to 30-millisecond intervals and 590 nm (total fluence, 45 J/cm^2) for the deeper vessels, followed within minutes by a single 2- to 5-millisecond pulse and 550-nm cutoff at 20 to 35 J/cm^2 fluence. Using this regimen, the immediate results are not always apparent because there is usually no purpura produced. Tissue erythema varies from mild to moderate.

Quasi–Continuous Wave Lasers

KTP (532 nm)

Medium- and large-caliber linear telangiectasias on the nose and cheeks are treated with either a 0.25- or 1-mm handpiece using average energies of 0.12 to 0.2 watts. Small, diffuse or mat telangiectasias can be treated with a 4-mm handpiece at average 0.7-watt energy. The laser beam is focused on the skin's surface in a noncontact mode. Immediate blanching of the vessels occurs with KTP laser irradiation, followed by mild erythema, edema, and crusting. Residual lesions can be retreated after 4 weeks.

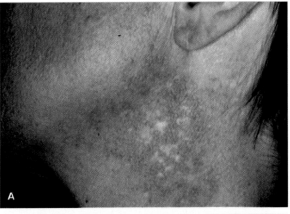

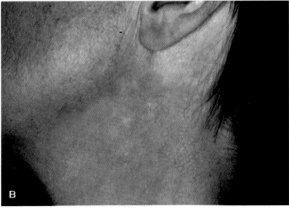

Figure 3-6

Poikiloderma on the neck of a 55-year-old woman before (*A*) and 8 weeks after (*B*) third treatment with the 585-nm pulsed dye laser at average fluence of 6 J/cm^2 using a 7-mm spot.

Krypton (568 nm)

Facial telangiectasias are treated using a 100-μm collimated handpiece at 0.4 to 0.6 watts with a 0.2-second pulse. Alternatively, a 1-mm handpiece can be used at 0.7 to 0.9 watts with a 0.2-second pulse. Treatment endpoints include lesional blanching with mild cutaneous erythema and edema.

Argon-Pumped Tunable Dye (577 to 585 nm)

Linear telangiectasias can be carefully traced with a spot size of 100 μm, low power of 0.1 to 0.4 watts, and pulses of 0.05 to 0.1 second to effect vessel disappearance. For small diffuse telangiectasias, a robotic hexagonal scanner (hexascan) is attached, and average fluences of 18 to 20 J/cm^2 are used with pulse widths of 30 to 100 milliseconds. When larger-caliber vessels are present, the hexagonal

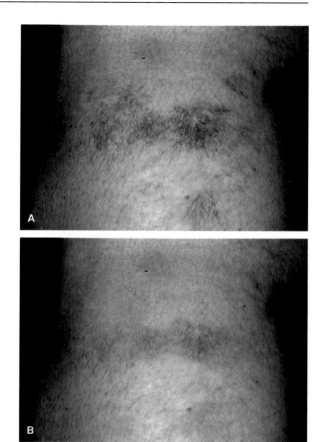

Figure 3-7
Spider veins and mat telangiectasias in the popliteal fossa of a 40-year-old woman before (A) and 6 weeks after (B) a single 595-nm long-pulse (1.5 ms) laser treatment at 20 J/cm^2.

scanner is used at fluences of 22 to 30 J/cm^2 and pulse widths of 30 to 100 milliseconds. Immediate blanching of the vessels is noted, with mild tissue hyperemia and swelling following irradiation.

Copper Vapor (578 nm)

Facial telangiectasias are typically treated using a 150-μm handpiece, pulse duration of 20 nanoseconds, repetition rate of 15 kHz, and average power of 0.35 to 0.55 watts delivered in 0.2-second exposure intervals using an electronic shuttering device. The laser handpiece is advanced along the vessel with each successive exposure. Visual magnification (3.5$\times$ to 6$\times$) is recommended to observe the vessel blanching endpoint. Mild swelling can occur within 24 hours, and mild crusting of the overlying skin appears within 3 days and resolves in 1 week. When necessary, repeat treatment can be delivered at 2 months.

► Summary

Multiple vascular-specific lasers are available to treat vascular lesions. Telangiectasias can be safely and effectively treated using any one of a wide variety of pulsed and quasi-CW lasers. Congenital lesions (port-wine stains, in particular) are best treated with a 585-nm pulsed dye laser because of its superior vascular specificity. Further developments in technology now suggest that laser treatment could be a viable option for leg telangiectasia, a condition previously treated by sclerotherapy alone. In addition, lesions recalcitrant or no longer responsive to pulsed dye laser treatment (such as certain port-wine stains) may achieve additional lightening using long-pulsed systems at vascular-specific wavelengths.

Manual of Cutaneous Laser Techniques, by Tina S. Alster.
Lippincott–Raven Publishers, Philadelphia © 1997.

CHAPTER 4

LASER TREATMENT OF PIGMENTED LESIONS

Lesion Categorization ▶ *Laser Treatment Options* ▶
Preoperative Patient Evaluation ▶ *Laser Treatment Protocol*

The concept of selective photothermolysis proposed by Anderson and Parrish in the early 1980s was first applied to the development of a laser for the treatment of vascular lesions (see Chap. 3) and was later put into practice in the development of a pigment-specific laser. Before this time, available lasers, such as the argon, CO_2, and Nd:YAG lasers, were used in a nonspecific manner to cauterize pigmented lesions. Because cutaneous pigment absorbs light at a wide spectrum of wavelengths (ranging from about 400 to 1000 nm), a multitude of different lasers can be used to treat pigmented lesions (Table 4-1).

The laser target is the melanosome, the cellular organelle that contains melanin. Its thermal relaxation time has been estimated at 10 to 100 nanoseconds, but any laser pulse width shorter than 1 microsecond can selectively damage a melanosome. Melanosomal damage is thought to occur from selective heating and from shock waves or cavitation by thermal expansion. Melanosomal alterations have been shown to be similar at various wavelengths, but they differ in terms of the threshold dose and depth of dermal penetration. In general, less energy is required to damage melanosomes using shorter wavelengths, whereas greater energy is needed to effect the same damage at longer wavelengths, owing to a decrease in the melanin absorption coefficient as wavelength increases. The advantage of lasers with longer wavelengths is their ability to affect deeper dermal pigment, whereas shorter-wavelength lasers can treat superficial epidermal pigment using lower energies.

TABLE 4-1. **PIGMENT-SPECIFIC LASERS**

Laser Type	Laser Specifics
Pulsed dye	510 nm, 300-ns pulse
Copper vapor	511 nm, quasi-CW
Krypton	520–530 nm, quasi-CW
KTP	532 nm, quasi-CW
Frequency-doubled Nd:YAG	532 nm, Q-switched
Q-switched ruby	694 nm, 25- to 40-ns pulse
Q-switched alexandrite	755 nm, 50- to 100-ns pulse
Q-switched Nd:YAG	1064 nm, 10- to 20-ns pulse

▶ Lesion Categorization

Before deciding which pigment-specific laser to use, you should determine whether the pigment in the lesion is primarily located superficially in the epidermis or deeper in the dermis (Table 4-2).

Epidermal Lesions

Lentigines

Lentigines are small, tan to medium brown macules that can arise on any skin surface or mucous membrane. They are usually smaller than 1 cm in diameter but can grow much larger. They usually arise in skin that has received excessive sun exposure and increase in number and size as a person ages. Lentigines may also be seen in association with a number of different cutaneous syndromes (eg, Peutz-Jeghers and LEOPARD syndromes). They should be differentiated from cutaneous malignancies, such as lentigo maligna and superficial spreading melanoma, on clinical or histologic grounds before laser treatment is begun.

TABLE 4-2. **CATEGORIZATION OF PIGMENTED LESIONS**

Epidermal	Dermal	Mixed
Lentigines	Nevi of Ota or Ito	Postinflammatory pigment
Ephelides	Melanocytic nevi	Melasma
Café-au-lait macule	Blue nevi	Nevus spilus
Becker's nevus		

Ephelides

Ephelides are freckles that appear as small, tan macules (usually 1 to 2 mm in diameter) on sun-exposed skin. They are most common in people with pale skin and blond to red hair and first appear in childhood after sun exposure.

Café-au-Lait Macules

Café-au-lait macules are typically light tan to light brown, flat macules or patches that are often first apparent at birth (or shortly thereafter). They range in size from 1 cm to 20 cm in diameter. They are seen in about 10% of the population, usually as solitary lesions, but are found in increased numbers in various syndromes, such as neurofibromatosis and Albright's syndrome.

Becker's Nevi

Becker's nevi are clinically similar to café-au-lait macules in that a light tan to brown patch is present, but they are more rare, occurring in about 0.5% of the population. They vary in size, but usually are large (ranging from 5 to 40 cm in diameter). The hyperpigmentation typically overlies a thickened dermis with enlarged bundles of smooth muscle (smooth muscle hamartoma). Coarse dark hairs are usually present within the patch, typically located over the deltoid or scapular regions.

Dermal Lesions

Nevi of Ota or Ito

A nevus of Ota clinically appears as a blue-gray patch on the face, usually unilateral, around the eye, temple, and cheek (areas innervated by the first and second branches of the trigeminal nerve). Ipsilateral scleral pigmentation is also commonly seen. Nevus of Ito displays the same type of blue-gray discoloration, but its location on the shoulder or upper arm indicate cutaneous areas innervated by the posterior supraclavicular and lateral brachial nerves. These lesions are most commonly seen in Asians; the incidence of nevi of Ota in Japanese is estimated to be 1% to 2% (nevi of Ito are much rarer). The distinctive skin discoloration is related to the deep placement of pigment, which imparts a bluish tone to the overlying skin as a result of the Tyndall effect of scattered light.

Melanocytic Nevi

Whether acquired or congenital, melanocytic nevi tend to appear as medium to dark brown macules; they can be located on any area of the body and range in size from 0.5 cm to several centimeters in diameter. The color of the nevus is related to the amount of pigment present and whether the pigment is located at the dermal–epidermal junction or in the superficial or deep dermis. Congenital melanocytic or nevocellular nevi occur in 1% to 2.5% of newborns and have been linked with a higher relative risk of melanoma (especially when they are very large). They tend to occur predominantly on the trunk and extremities.

Blue Nevi

A blue nevus is usually solitary and appears as a blue-black, well-circumscribed papule less than 1 cm in diameter. It arises spontaneously in children and young adults and is twice as common in men as in women. The blue color is related to the light-scattering effect (Tyndall effect) of the tissue overlying the deeply placed dermal pigment.

Mixed Lesions

Postinflammatory Hyperpigmentation

This tan to medium brown pigmentation can arise in any area of skin that has been traumatized (usually by blunt, sharp, or thermal cutaneous injury or by photodamage). It is most commonly seen in people with darker skin tones but can arise in any skin type. The mechanism by which this pigmentation occurs is not fully understood, but in the case of traumatic injury through the dermal–epidermal junction, melanin incontinence occurs, with subsequent displacement of melanin into the superficial or deep dermis.

Melasma

Melasma is a light to medium brown symmetric facial discoloration. It is an acquired condition that is most commonly associated with pregnancy or oral contraceptive use. Like postinflammatory hyperpigmentation, its cause is unknown, but two basic types of melasma exist. The epidermal type shows deposition of melanin in the basal or suprabasal layers of the epidermis, whereas the dermal type exhibits additional melanophages in the superficial and deep dermis. The fact that the pigmentation is usually located in the sun-exposed areas of the face (cheeks and forehead, in particular) is suggestive of additional etiologic factors.

Nevus Spilus

Nevus spilus is characterized by what appears clinically as a café-au-lait spot containing darker brown speckles. The darker areas are histologically consistent with either junctional or compound nevi, whereas the tan portions relate to an increase of melanocytes and hyperpigmentation in the rete ridges. This lesion is usually seen on the trunk and extremities and occurs in about 2% of the population.

▶ Laser Treatment Options

As discussed earlier, there are several pigment-specific lasers from which to choose for treating pigmented lesions (Table 4-3). Your ultimate decision should be based on the type of pigmented lesion (superficial or deep) and the known response rates of pigmented lesions to various lasers. Even though cutaneous pigment can absorb light at many different wavelengths, pigment may not clear as efficiently as you might expect in actual clinical practice. This is due to the fact that a lased

TABLE 4-3. **RESPONSES OF PIGMENTED LESIONS TO LASER TREATMENT**

Laser Type	Ephelides, Lentigines	Café-au-Lait	Nevus of Ota	Benign nevi	Melasma PIH	Nevus spilus	Becker's nevus
Pulsed dye	+ + +	+ + +	0	+	0	+ /0	+ /0
Copper vapor	+ +	+	0	+	0	Unknown	Unknown
Krypton	+ +	+ /0	0	+	0	Unknown	Unknown
KTP	+ +	Unknown	0	+	0	Unknown	Unknown
Frequency-doubled Nd:YAG	+ + +	+ +	0	+	0	+ /0	+ /0
QS ruby	+ + +	+ /+ +	+ + +	+ +	0	+ /0	+ /0
QS alexandrite	+ +	+	+ + +	+ +	0	+ /0	+ /0
QS Nd:YAG	+ +	+ /0	+ + +	+ +	0	+ /0	+ /0

0, no effect; +, fair; + +, good; + + +, excellent; PIH, postinflammatory hyperpigmentation; QS, Q-switched.

area normally repigments from the residual melanocytes in the adjacent skin and by adnexal structures in the area. In addition, mild stimulation of melanogenesis can occur, especially when treating such lesions as melasma and postinflammatory hyperpigmentation. Therefore, laser treatment of pigmented lesions can be difficult. I routinely tell patients with café-au-lait spots and other pigmented lesions that they are, by far, the hardest to treat because of the unpredictable nature of pigment response. Because of the fact that melasma and postinflammatory hyperpigmentation both tend to recur or worsen after *any* type of pigment-specific laser irradiation, I avoid treating these lesions with laser.

Pulsed and Quality-Switched Lasers

The 510-nm pulsed dye laser with a 300-nanosecond pulse duration is the prototypic pulsed laser used in the treatment of superficial pigmented lesions, such as lentigines and café-au-lait macules. Its short wavelength and pulse duration are aptly suited for maximal epidermal pigment absorption with decreased risk of untoward dermal reaction.

Quality-switched (Q-switched) systems, whereby ultrashort bursts (10 to 100 nanoseconds) of stored high energy are produced, include the 694-nm ruby laser, the 755-nm alexandrite laser, and the 1064-nm Nd:YAG laser. The longer wavelengths of these lasers make them most suitable for the treatment of dermal pigmented lesions, such as nevi of Ota. Superficial or epidermal pigmented lesions can also be treated, but at the risk of greater unwanted dermal damage, especially when only a small amount of epidermal pigment is present.

Quasi–Continuous Wave Lasers

A few quasi–continuous wave (CW) lasers (eg, krypton, KTP, copper vapor) are used to treat cutaneous pigmented lesions. Their wavelengths range from 510 nm to 532 nm; these shorter, green wavelengths are used to eliminate primarily epidermal pigment. As such, these quasi-CW lasers are best used for ephelides and lentigines. Their use in café-au-lait spots is limited because of the excessive heat that they produce in the normal tissue, resulting from the prolonged pulses or trains of pulses that exceed the thermal relaxation time of a melanosome. The short wavelengths with limited tissue penetration preclude them from being highly effective in the treatment of dermal pigmented lesions, such as nevi of Ota.

▶ Preoperative Patient Evaluation

Patients present for possible laser treatment of pigmented lesions ranging from a few scattered lentigines to large café-au-lait spots and congenital nevi. You should determine whether the presenting lesion would be amenable to the current laser technology and whether you have the skill to treat it. In addition to the issues raised in Chapter 2, some special considerations pertinent to pigmented lesion treatment follow.

Does the patient have a pigmented lesion that can be adequately treated with laser surgery?

Café-au-lait spots and nevi of Ota are particularly suited for laser treatment because any other treatment, such as excision or cryotherapy (which have been widely used for these lesions in the past), usually produce significant scarring. Patients with café-au-lait spots, in particular, need to know that some lesions may not be responsive to laser treatment for unknown reasons, or they may recur after the lesion was thought to have been eradicated.

Patients with solar lentigines and ephelides have other treatment options that they can consider that yield fair to excellent results, including cryotherapy, the use of bleaching agents, and chemical peels. The pigment within melanocytic nevi can be selectively targeted by any one of the Q-switched laser systems; however, laser treatment of these lesions remains controversial because of their premalignant potential. On the one hand, a reduction of lesional pigment (malignant precursors) by laser irradiation could potentially decrease this risk, but on the other hand, removal of pigment within a lesion could decrease the ability to detect a malignant melanoma. Although no proof exists, repeated laser injury to residual nevus cells may predispose to malignant change.

Melasma and postinflammatory hyperpigmentation are not amenable to pigment-specific laser treatment of *any* type. These pigmented lesions have a tendency to recur or worsen after laser irradiation for reasons that remain unclear. My hypothesis is that the laser impact on the tissue in these lesions may be interpreted as an injury, resulting in further postinflammatory hyperpigmentation.

Has the patient undergone previous treatment to the lesion?

Many patients with lentigines have received treatment with a number of over-the-counter and prescription fading creams or with cryotherapy. Unless the previous cryotherapy resulted in tissue fibrosis, the pigment-specific laser treatment can be delivered without difficulty. If fibrosis or hypopigmentation exists, patients need to be aware that laser eradication of the lesion may be more difficult. Similarly, café-au-lait macules or nevi of Ota that have undergone other forms of treatment, producing some degree of fibrosis or scar, may require additional treatments to obtain the desired degree of lightening.

Does the patient or another family member have a history of melanoma?

Although no known cases of malignant transformation have occurred within a benign pigmented lesion as a consequence of laser irradiation, it is wise to be aware of the familial potential and to document accordingly. In one reported case, a lentigo maligna treated with an argon laser in the early 1980s revealed absence of melanocytic hyperplasia 8 months after treatment, but the malignancy recurred 4 years after the original treatment.

What is the patient's skin type?

Patients with darker skin tones are more difficult to treat because the pigment-specific laser light targets the most accessible pigment first. That means that a dermal pigmented lesion in a patient with darker skin may have less lesional pigment removed because of the competing overlying chromophores (melanosomes) in the epidermis. The patient should be warned of the possibility of hypopigmentation (usually transient) due to destruction of these melanosomes and also be prepared for additional laser treatments if the laser light cannot penetrate the deeper dermis efficiently.

Does the patient have realistic expectations of the laser treatment?

Lentigines typically require only one or two laser treatments to achieve clearance. More extensive pigmented lesions, such as café-au-lait macules and nevi of Ota, always require additional treatments (Table 4-4). A patient with a Becker's nevus or nevus spilus should be cautioned that these types of lesions are often unresponsive to laser treatment. Similarly, patients with café-au-lait spots should be encouraged but also forewarned that not all café-au-lait spots respond and that some may recur. Patients affected with melasma or postinflammatory hyperpigmentation should be strongly discouraged from pursuing laser treatment because of the high

TABLE 4-4. LASER TREATMENT OF PIGMENTED LESIONS: CLINICAL RESPONSE

Lesion	Number of Laser Treatments	Comments
Lentigines	1–3	
Ephilides	1–2	
Café-au-lait macules	2–10	May recur; occasionally unresponsive
Becker's nevus	2–6	Often unresponsive
Nevus of Ota or Ito	4–6	
Melanocytic nevi	2–6	
Nevus spilus	4–6	Often unresponsive
Melasma	N/A	Uniformly unresponsive
Postinflammatory pigment	N/A	Uniformly unresponsive

LASER TREATMENT OF PIGMENTED LESIONS: PREOPERATIVE CHECKLIST

Type of pigmented lesion:

_____ lentigines	_____ nevus of Ota/Ito
_____ ephelides	_____ melanocytic nevus
_____ café-au-lait macule	_____ postinflammatory pigment
_____ Becker's nevus	_____ melasma
_____ nevus spilus	_____ other (_____)

Location of lesion:

_____ scalp	_____ arms	_____ back
_____ face	_____ legs	_____ abdomen
_____ neck	_____ hands	_____ buttocks
_____ chest	_____ feet	_____ other (_____)

Prior treatment (list with dates): _____

Personal or family history of melanoma (yes/no) or dysplastic nevi (yes/no)
If yes, list with dates/treatment received: _____

Medical problems (list): _____

Current medications: _____

Allergies: _____

Instruction sheet given to patient and thoroughly reviewed _____ (initials/date)

Patient instructed to wear sunscreen, avoid sun exposure, and to *not tan*
    during course of laser treatment _____ (initials/date)

Informed consent reviewed and signed _____ (initials/date)

Preoperative photographs taken _____ (initials/date)

First laser treatment scheduled (type/date) _____

Postoperative skin care reviewed and written instructions given to
    patient _____ (initials/date)

LASER TREATMENT OF PIGMENTED LESIONS: INFORMED CONSENT

I, _____, understand that I have a benign pigmented lesion called a _____. Dr. _____ has explained to me that although laser surgery is effective in most cases, no guarantees can be made that I will benefit from treatment. I understand that several treatment sessions may be needed to obtain the desired level of improvement. Sometimes, a lesion will not completely clear but will become lighter; occasionally, a pigmented lesion may not respond to laser treatment at all.

The most common side effects and complications of this laser treatment are as follows:

1. *Pain.* The snapping and burning sensation of each laser pulse may produce a minimal to moderate amount of discomfort. An anesthetic cream or injection may be used to block the pain if desired.
2. *Bruising.* Immediately after the laser treatment, the area will appear white, then turn purplish in color like a bruise. The discoloration will fade during the next 7 to 10 days.
3. *Swelling.* Areas most likely to swell are under the eyes and neck. The swelling subsides within 3 to 5 days with regular ice application.
4. *Blisters or scabs.* These can also develop and can take 1 to 2 weeks to resolve.
5. *Skin darkening (hyperpigmentation).* This can occur in the treated areas and will fade within 2 to 6 months. This reaction is more common in patients with olive or dark skin tones and can worsen if the laser-treated area is exposed to the sun.
6. *Skin lightening (hypopigmentation).* This can occur in an area of skin that has already received several treatments. The light spots usually darken or repigment in 3 to 6 months but can be permanent in rare cases.
7. *Scarring.* This is extremely rare after pigment-specific laser therapy, but can occur on disruption of the skin's surface. Following all advised postoperative instructions will reduce the possibility of this occurrence.
8. *Lesion persistence or recurrence.* Some pigmented lesions may not go away completely or may recur after treatment despite the best efforts made by the doctor.

I further understand that, if left untreated, my pigmented lesion would not be expected to go away on its own. It also would not pose a medical threat, but could become darker and larger with time.

By providing my signature below, I acknowledge that I have read and understood all of the information written above and feel that I have been adequately informed of my alternative treatment options, the risks of the proposed laser surgery, and the risks of not treating my condition. I hereby freely consent to the laser surgery to be performed by Dr. _____ and authorize the taking of clinical photographs, which will be used solely for my medical records unless my physician deems that their anonymous use (in lectures or scientific publications) could benefit medical research and education. They will not be used for advertising without my written permission.

_____   _____
Patient's or Guardian's Signature   Date   Witness' Signature   Date

rate of lesional recurrence or worsening. These patients often are frustrated with the lack of laser treatment options, and they should be further evaluated for more aggressive topical treatment or chemical peel.

A checklist that remains in the patient's medical record is helpful during the initial evaluation of a patient with a pigmented lesion who desires laser treatment. If the patient is found to be a suitable candidate for pigment-specific laser treatment, the proper information sheet (see Chap. 2) and verbal explanations are provided. Once informed consent has been obtained, baseline preoperative photographs are taken, and the patient is ready for laser treatment.

▶ Laser Treatment Protocol

An intraoperative checklist and patient treatment log help to prevent oversights and ensure proper procedural documentation. Operative reports are helpful in cases in which insurance reimbursement is sought, such as in patients with pigmented birthmarks, which qualify as congenital lesions for insurance purposes.

LASER TREATMENT OF PIGMENTED LESIONS: OPERATIVE CHECKLIST

▶ Pigmented laser in ''ready'' mode and calibrated to correct energy with proper handpiece
▶ Anesthetic cream or makeup completely removed with mild soap and water
▶ Safety goggles or glasses on operating personnel and patient
▶ No flammable substances in operating area
▶ Hair protected with wet gauze or headband
▶ Tissues and ice water available for patient comfort
▶ Hand-held fan to cool patient during treatment
▶ Laser tray: bacitracin, polysporin, or mupirocin (Bactroban) ointment, wet gauze, ice pack, Telfa pad, Vigilon, or other wound dressing, cotton swabs
▶ Written postoperative instructions given to patient
▶ Return appointment scheduled

LASER TREATMENT OF PIGMENTED LESIONS: TREATMENT LOG

Patient name: _____ Age: _____

Skin type: _____

Diagnosis:_____

Previous treatment(s): _____

    Treatment #_____   Photos taken: yes/no

    Date: _____

    Laser used: _____

    Fluence or power: _____ (J/cm^2 or watts)

    Spot size: _____

    Anesthesia: _____

    Tissue cooling: yes/no

    Location treated: _____

    Area (in cm) treated: _____

    Number of laser pulses: _____

    Total treatment time: _____

    Skin appearance S/P rx: _____

    Complications: _____

    Bacitracin/Telfa pad/Vigilon applied: yes/no

    Return appointment scheduled: _____ (date)

    Home care: bacitracin/Telfa pad/acetaminophen (circle)

LASER TREATMENT OF PIGMENTED LESIONS: SAMPLE OPERATIVE REPORT

Patient name: _____

Diagnosis: _____

Date of operation: _____

Surgeon: _____

Procedure performed: Treatment of _____ [lesion] of

the _____ [location] with the _____

laser

Anesthesia: _____

Total anesthesia time: _____

Laser Procedure

The patient was brought into the operating room and placed in a supine position. Protective goggles were placed on the patient, and hair-bearing areas were protected. The _____ laser was calibrated to _____ [energy], and the _____ [lesion] of the _____ [location] (total area of _____ cm) was treated with a _____-mm spot size. The laser-irradiated area(s) showed the expected ash-white tissue response. The patient tolerated the procedure well.

Total operative time: _____

Postoperative wound dressings: Bacitracin ointment/Telfa pad/Vigilon

Postoperative medications: acetaminophen _____ mg orally every 4 to 6 hours as needed

Postoperative disposition of patient: stable and ambulatory

Follow-up appointment scheduled: 6 to 8 weeks

Surgeon's signature   Date

Pulsed Dye (510 nm)

Epidermal pigmented lesions, such as lentigines and café-au-lait spots, respond well to 510-nm pulsed dye laser irradiation (Figs. 4-1 to 4-3). Treatments are usually initiated at 2 to 3 J/cm^2 using nonoverlapping 5-mm laser spots, which produce an immediate ash-white tissue response. If pinpoint bleeding or epidermal rupture occurs on laser impact, the fluence should be decreased by 0.25 J/cm^2 or more until the desired ash-white skin response is observed. Response to treatment is determined at 6 to 8 weeks, which allows for adequate cutaneous healing in most cases. If postinflammatory hyperpigmented laser spots are observed within the treated lesion at the time of follow-up, a bleaching cream, such as hydroquinone, combined with glycolic or retinoic acid is prescribed for daily topical use until the spots resolve (Fig. 4-4). If only residual lesional pigment is present on follow-up examination, another laser treatment can be delivered at the same or slightly increased fluence.

Lentigines do not repigment when treatment intervals are prolonged, but café-au-lait macules have been known to darken from residual lesional pigment or from neighboring follicular appendages. Proper timing of laser treatments for café-au-lait macules, with fine fluence adjustments made as indicated by lesional

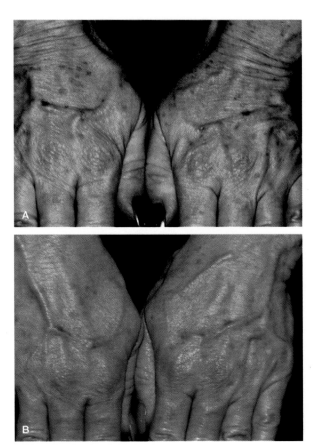

Figure 4-1

Solar lentigines on the dorsal hands of a 55-year-old woman before (*A*) and 6 weeks after (*B*) one treatment using a 510-nm pulsed dye laser at 2.5 J/cm^2 and 5-mm spot size.

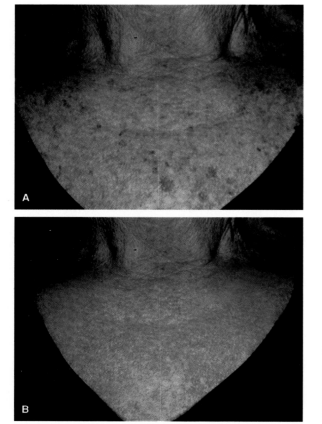

Figure 4-2
A 70-year-old woman with multiple lentigines on her chest before (*A*) and after (*B*) two treatments with a 510-nm pulsed dye laser at average fluence of 2.25 J/cm² using a 5-mm spot size.

response to each treatment, is necessary to maximize the effect of treatment and to avoid recurrence. Every last remnant of lesional pigment within the café-au-lait macule must be treated to reduce the risk of recurrence. Lentigines generally require only 1 or 2 laser treatments, whereas café-au-lait macules are highly variable; they may clear with as few as 2 or 3 treatments or only after as many as 10 or 12 treatments (average, 8 to 9). Some café-au-lait macules remain totally unresponsive to treatment.

Copper Vapor (511 nm)

The copper vapor laser is used at average powers of 0.16 to 0.25 watts to treat lentigines. Typically, lentigines clear within one or two treatment sessions using a 150-μm spot at 0.2-second intervals. Response of café-au-lait macules has been highly variable, with reports of textural changes and scarring within irradiated lesions.

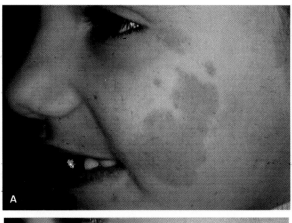

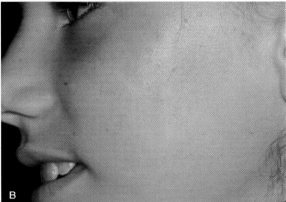

Figure 4-3

Café-au-lait birthmark in a 10-year-old girl before (A) and 4 months after (B) eight laser treatments with the 510-nm pulsed dye laser at average fluence of 2.75 J/cm^2 using a 5-mm spot size.

Krypton (520 to 530 nm)

The krypton laser is essentially used to treat lentigines. It is generally operated at 700 mW with a 0.2-second pulse and a 1-mm handpiece.

Frequency-Doubled Nd : YAG (532 nm)

Solar lentigines and café-au-lait macules are typically treated at fluences of 2 to 2.5 J/cm^2, with 1- to 3-mm spot sizes, and at rates of 10 Hz. Lentigines can easily be eliminated within one or two laser sessions, whereas café-au-lait spots are highly variable in terms of pigment responses and rates of recurrence. As has also been observed with 510-nm pulsed dye treatment, the frequency-doubled Nd : YAG laser can sometimes be successful in totally eradicating a café-au-lait macule, or it may fail to remove any significant pigment. Lesional recurrence after complete clinical clearing has also been reported. The reasons for this are unclear but probably relate more to the nature of café-au-lait macules than to the pigment specificity of any laser.

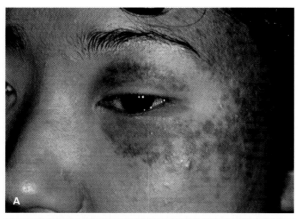

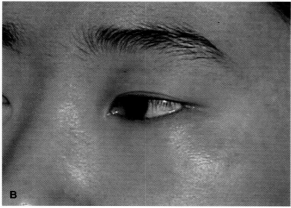

Figure 4-4

A 20-year-old woman with a nevus of Ota before (*A*) and 6 months after (*B*) her sixth treatment with the QS alexandrite laser (755 nm, 100 ns) at average fluence of 6.5 J/cm^2 and 3-mm spot size.

Q-Switched Ruby (694 nm)

Epidermal and dermal pigmented lesions can be treated using the ruby laser at fluences of 5 to 6 J/cm^2. Lentigines are cleared within one or two treatments, whereas responsive café-au-lait macules require four or more treatments at bimonthly intervals. Dermal melanocytic lesions, such as nevi of Ota, can be cleared within an average of four to six treatments. It does not appear important to eliminate all lesional pigment (as with café-au-lait macules) to prevent recurrence. Infraorbital hyperpigmentation can be lightened significantly after one or two laser sessions.

Q-Switched Alexandrite (755 nm)

The tissue effects of Q-switched alexandrite laser are similar to those obtained with the ruby laser. The alexandrite laser treats dermal pigment better than epidermal pigment; thus, café-au-lait macules and lentigines are not as effectively treated as nevi of Ota and melanocytic nevi. Fluences of 6 to 7 J/cm^2 are typically used

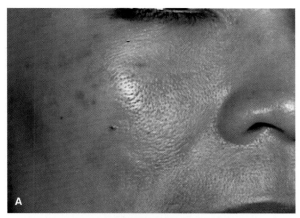

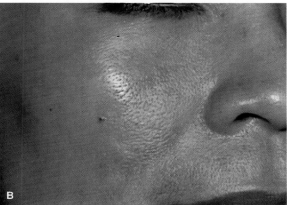

Figure 4-5

A 32-year-old woman with malar hyperpigmentation before (*A*) and 4 months after (*B*) one 510-nm pulsed dye laser treatment at 2.5 J/cm^2. The laser-treated areas initially hyperpigmented after treatment and resolved only with the use of topical hydroquinone and glycolic acid creams.

with a 3-mm spot size at 6- to 8-week intervals. An ash-white tissue response is observed on laser impact. An average of five or six treatments are needed to clear nevus of Ota, whereas three treatments have produced significant clinical and histologic clearing of melanocytic nevi (Fig. 4-5). Two laser sessions at 6 J/cm^2 have also been reported to lighten infraorbital hyperpigmentation significantly.

Q-Switched Nd:YAG (1064 nm)

The longer wavelength of the Nd:YAG laser permits deeper dermal penetration, thus maximizing its suitability for treatment of dermal pigmented lesions. Nevi of Ota require an average of five laser treatments at 8 J/cm^2 using a 3-mm spot size. Similar parameters are used to treat benign melanocytic nevi.

▶ Summary

A number of pigment-specific lasers are available that can effectively treat a variety of epidermal and dermal pigmented lesions without complication because melanin can absorb light at a wide range of visible wavelengths. Certain pigmented lesions remain difficult to predict in terms of their ability to be treated, the possibility of recurrence (eg, café-au-lait spots, nevus spilus), or their unresponsiveness (eg, melasma, postinflammatory hyperpigmentation). Further investigations are needed to determine the reasons for such variable clinical responses in lesions that, histologically, appear similar. Unfortunately, melasma and postinflammatory hyperpigmentation, two common dermatologic problems, remain unresponsive to laser treatment.

Manual of Cutaneous Laser Techniques, by Tina S. Alster.
Lippincott–Raven Publishers, Philadelphia © 1997.

CHAPTER **5**

LASER TREATMENT OF TATTOOS

Tattoo Categorization ▶ *Laser Treatment Options* ▶
Preoperative Patient Evaluation ▶ *Laser Treatment
Protocol*

Tattoos have been in existence since the Stone Age, and their popularity appears to be on the rise. More than 10 million people in the United States have at least one tattoo. Despite their rise in popularity, more than half the people with tattoos eventually regret having had them placed. Attempts at their removal date back to Egyptian mummies, who showed evidence of partial tattoo removal. Fortunately for those with undesirable tattoos in present day, there are now lasers that can effectively remove tattoos without the adverse sequelae so commonly encountered with previous treatments. Scar formation or pigmentary alteration, which was almost as undesirable as the original tattoo, was commonly seen after treatments such as dermabrasion, salabrasion, surgical excision, and cryosurgery. The development of quality-switched (Q-switched, or QS) lasers, which use ultrashort pulses in the nanosecond range and high energies to shatter tattoo ink particles have enabled laser surgeons to treat unwanted tattoos safely and effectively. Although the mechanism is not fully understood, tattoo ink removal is probably facilitated by the lymphatic clearing of tattoo particles, which are blasted free from tissue macrophages on laser impact. Clinical improvement also occurs as a result of a change in tissue optical properties after laser irradiation.

Because of the multiple ink colors, various compositions of dyes used, and the different types of tattoos that can be obtained, response to laser treatment is anything but uniform. To determine the best laser (or lasers) for the job, it is crucial to determine the type of tattoo present, with careful consideration of its pigment composition.

TABLE 5-1. **TATTOO CATEGORIZATION**

Tattoo Types	Pigment Type	Ink Concentration	Pigment Depth
Professional	Organometallic dyes	Dense	Deep
Amateur	India ink (carbon)	Sparse	Variable
Cosmetic	Iron or titanium oxide	Sparse	Superficial
Traumatic	Carbon, metals, dirt	Variable	Variable
Medicinal	India ink (carbon)	Sparse	Superficial

▶ Tattoo Categorization

Tattoos can be broadly categorized into the types listed in Table 5-1 and described in the following sections.

Professional Tattoos

These tattoos are "professionally" placed using hand-held tattoo guns by tattoo artists and are composed of one or several colors of organometallic dyes. Uniformly deep dermal injections of large amounts of ink account for the clear, sharp, strong clinical images of these tattoos. Localized cutaneous and rare systemic allergic reactions to colored inks have been reported, most commonly to red (mercury), yellow (cadmium), green (chromium), and blue (cobalt). With time, the colors may fade (especially the reds and yellows), and the tattoo borders and lines blur and become indistinct as a result of the movement of pigment even deeper into the dermis and to the progressive clearing of pigment by the lymphatic system to regional nodes. Older tattoos, therefore, take on a blue-gray, blurred appearance, with a variable amount of colored pigment intact.

Amateur Tattoos

Usually etched into the skin by a friend or even by the patient, an amateur tattoo appears gray or blue-black in color. Simple carbon or India ink is used. A variable amount of tattoo ink is injected at variable depths into the skin. The resultant tattoo is not typically as sharp and well defined as its professionally placed counterpart because of the relative paucity of injected ink and the lack of bright colors used.

Cosmetic Tattoos

Lipliner, eyeliner, and eyebrow tattoos are becoming more common, and the boutique business is flourishing with women who no longer desire spending 30 or more minutes daily putting on makeup. Usually brown, black, and red inks composed of iron or titanium oxide are used to create the appropriate cosmetic liner. They are typically placed free-hand by a cosmetologist specially trained in their application (although it is a totally unregulated practice).

Traumatic Tattoos

Traumatic tattoos result from mechanical penetration of the skin by such foreign body particles as metal, glass, dirt, and carbon-containing material. A combination of skin abrasion and impregnation by pigmented particles occurs as a result of trauma involving friction with road surfaces or blast injuries. Depending on the extent of injury, the substances can become so deeply embedded in the skin that their removal is extremely difficult.

Medicinal Tattoos

Small tattoos may be placed by medical personnel to mark ports for radiation treatment or catheter placement. They appear as gray or blue-black spots measuring 1 to 3 mm in diameter and can serve as a vivid and unwelcome reminder to patients of their unpleasant treatment and ultimate mortality.

▶ Laser Treatment Options

Several tattoo-specific lasers are available for treatment. Your ultimate selection should be determined by the type of tattoo and ink colors present. Different lasers can treat different colored pigments (Table 5-2). Unfortunately, no single laser can adequately clear all colors and types of tattoo ink. So, if you are serious about treating tattoos, you must resign yourself to having more than one tattoo-specific laser at your disposal.

TABLE 5-2. **RESPONSE OF TATTOO INKS TO LASER TREATMENT**

Laser Type	Parameters	Response			
		Black Ink	Green Ink	Red Ink	Tan Ink
Pulsed dye	510 nm, 300 ns	Poor	Poor	Excellent	May blacken
Frequency-doubled Nd:YAG	532 nm, 10–40 ns	Poor	Poor	Excellent	Usually blackens
QS ruby	694 nm, 25–50 ns	Excellent	Good	Poor	Usually blackens
QS alexandrite	755 nm, 50–100 ns	Excellent	Excellent	Poor	Usually blackens
QS Nd:YAG	1064 nm, 10 ns	Excellent	Fair	Poor	Usually blackens

Modified from Alster TS, Lewis AB. Dermatologic laser surgery: a review. Dermatol Surg 1996;22:797.

Quality-Switched Lasers

Quality-switched lasers are designed to produce a singular 10- to 100-nanosecond pulse with peak energies of up to 10 J/cm^2. This is accomplished by building up energy within the laser tube by the placement of a switch that denies photons access. When the switch is released, the millions of watts in power that have been generated and stored are emitted in a single high-energy pulse of light. The mechanism of action of a Q-switched laser system is through photon absorption by tattoo pigment–laden fibroblasts, producing temperatures greater than 1000°C. The immediate skin whitening observed on Q-switched laser impact probably represents rapid localized tissue heating with steam or gas formation, which produces epidermal and dermal vacuolization. The fragmentation of pigment-containing cells is thought to result from rapid thermal expansion, shock waves, and cavitation.

Ruby

Ruby lasers emit visible red light at 694 nm. The first laser ever built was a (non–Q-switched) ruby laser in 1960; soon thereafter, Goldman used the ruby laser to treat tattoos. Early evidence suggested that shorter pulses (in the nanosecond range) were needed to remove tattoo pigment more effectively. The technology was found to be impractical because only small areas could be treated at one time, and the high energies needed to effect more complete tattoo removal were causing too much collateral tissue damage. It took another 20 years before the ruby laser experienced a revival, and it was only then that its benefits were appreciated. It was found that although multiple laser treatments were generally necessary to effectively remove blue-black ink, tattoo removal could be accomplished with minimal risk of scarring. Many subsequent reports have validated the ruby laser's effectiveness and safety profile. In addition, further evidence suggests more rapid tattoo clearing and, therefore, fewer treatments when even shorter pulse durations (ie, 25 rather than 40 nanoseconds) are used. The ability to remove other colored inks varies with the ruby laser. Green tattoo ink can usually be eliminated, but red tattoo ink cannot.

Alexandrite

The alexandrite laser has a wavelength of 755 nm and a pulse duration of 50 to 100 nanoseconds. The light is delivered through a fiberoptic system with a 3-mm spot at 1 Hz. The alexandrite laser is the newest Q-switched system; it has been available on the market only since the early 1990s. Subsequent clinical and histologic reports have confirmed its ability to treat tattoos with the same degree of effectiveness as the QS ruby and QS Nd:YAG lasers (Figs. 5-1 and 5-2). Its advantage appears to lie in its ability to produce less tissue destruction (ie, tissue debris) during laser impact, so that fewer side effects (eg, hypopigmentation and textural change) are encountered. Multiple treatments remain necessary to achieve tattoo clearance with this laser, but green pigment can be cleared more effectively than with either the ruby or Nd:YAG systems (Figs. 5-3 and 5-4).

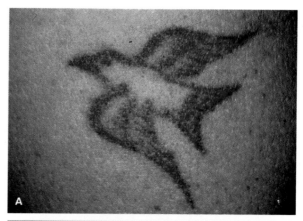

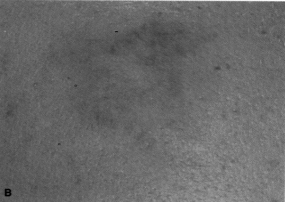

Figure 5-1

A 15-year-old professional tattoo with blue, black, and red inks on the arm of a 33-year-old man before (*A*) and 8 weeks after (*B*) eight laser treatments with a Q-switched alexandrite laser at average fluence of 6.5 J/cm^2 and 3-mm spot size. The red portion was eliminated after two 510-nm pulsed dye laser sessions at 3 J/cm^2 using a 5-mm spot.

Nd:YAG

The QS Nd:YAG laser has a wavelength of 1064 nm and pulse duration of 10 nanoseconds, which can be delivered with a 1.5- to 3-mm spot size at a repetition rate of up to 10 Hz. Its longer wavelength was initially thought to be more advantageous for tattoo removal because of its decreased absorption by melanin and ability for deeper dermal penetration. Although postoperative hypopigmentation was decreased using this system (especially in comparison with the ruby laser), its ability to remove tattoo pigment was no more effective than the other Q-switched laser systems. Blue-black tattoos can be cleared after several treatments, but green and red inks cannot be treated effectively at the 1064-nm wavelength.

Green-Light Lasers

Pulsed Dye

At a 510-nm wavelength and 300-nanosecond pulse duration, this pulsed dye system has been shown to be highly effective in the treatment of red, orange, and yellow tattoo inks. The number of treatments needed to result in red or yellow

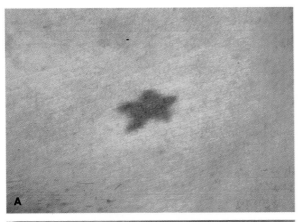

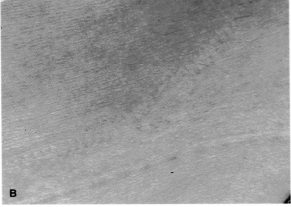

Figure 5-2

Amateur tattoo on the abdomen of a 36-year-old woman of 10 years' duration before (A) and 4 weeks after (B) fourth Q-switched alexandrite laser treatment at average fluence of 6.25 J/cm².

tattoo ink removal is less (average, two to four) than that needed by any of the aforementioned QS lasers to treat blue, black, or green pigments. The light is delivered through a flexible fiberoptic system with a 5-mm spot at 1 Hz.

Frequency-Doubled Nd:YAG

With the use of a crystal, the frequency of the 1064-nm Nd:YAG laser can be doubled, which effectively halves the wavelength to 532 nm. The 10-nanosecond pulse is delivered at up to 10 Hz through a 1.5- to 3-mm spot. As with the 510-nm pulsed dye laser, this system can treat red and sometimes yellow tattoo pigment within two to four treatment sessions.

Of special note is the inability of any of the aforementioned lasers to treat fleshtone (or tan) tattoos. These iron or titanium oxide–containing pigments are typically found in cosmetic tattoos but have been uncovered in tattoos that have been overtattooed for camouflage purposes. They can also be seen in certain brown and rust-colored inks used in decorative tattoos. All of these lasers have been reported to cause an immediate blackening reaction within the tattoo on laser impact. This reaction is believed to be due to reduction of ferric oxide (Fe_2O_3)—a

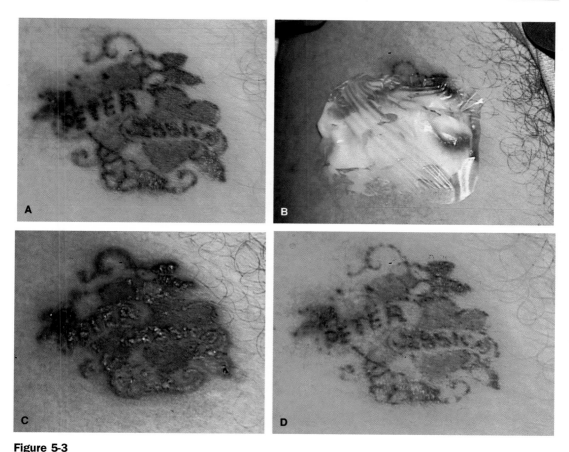

Figure 5-3

(A) Multicolored professional tattoo that had received two prior treatments with a Q-switched ruby laser. There is persistence of red pigment and blurring and fading of blue-black and green tattoo inks. (B) Same tattoo with 30% lidocaine USP in Velvachol cream under Tegaderm occlusion for 30 minutes before laser procedure. (C) Immediately after laser treatment using both the Q-switched alexandrite laser (for blue, black, and green inks) and 510-nm pulsed dye laser (for red inks). Note the absence of bleeding and fast-resolving ash-white tissue response with hyperemia. (D) Six weeks afterward, all tattoo colors have faded.

rust color—to ferrous oxide (FeO)—black. Unfortunately, it is impossible to predict which cosmetic inks will darken and whether further QS laser irradiation could reverse the tattoo darkening.

▶ Preoperative Patient Evaluation

Patients with tattoos represent all walks of life. No longer are images of back-alley tattoo parlors appropriate. Indeed, fashionable tattoo boutiques are cropping up in record numbers, and more people than ever are having decorative and cosmetic tattoos placed.

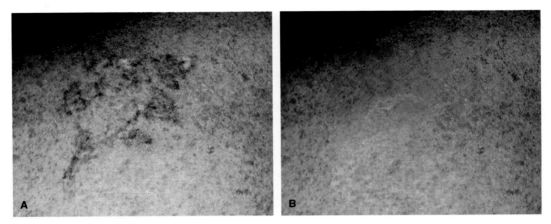

Figure 5-4
(A) Professional tattoo on the shoulder of a 37-year-old man who had received six prior treatments with the Q-switched Nd:YAG laser (1064 nm). There is persistence of green ink. (B) After four additional treatments with a QS alexandrite laser (755 nm, 50 to 100 ns, 3-mm spot size, average fluence 6.5 J/cm^2), the green ink was completely eliminated.

As stated earlier, however, most patients who are initially thrilled with their tattoos eventually live to regret them. Several questions relating to the tattoo must be answered before initiating treatment to ascertain which laser (if any) is most appropriate.

What type of tattoo is present?

Because different types of inks are used for different tattoos (see Fig. 5-1), and their eventual responses to different lasers vary, it is extremely important to determine whether the tattoo was placed by an amateur or professional. Professional tattoos are typically harder to remove because of deeper and denser tattoo pigment placement and the use of multiple colors of organometallic dyes (Fig. 5-5). Traumatic tattoos may require one, two, or several treatments because of the variable amount or depth of pigment involved.

Is the tattoo multicolored?

Tattoos with various ink colors are more difficult to remove. Typically, more than one laser is necessary to remove such common colors as green and red, each seen in about 30% of tattoos.

Does the tattoo contain tan, brown, rust, or white inks?

These colors are often used in cosmetic tattoos to add a permanent line around the mouth (lipliner), eyes (eyeliner), or eyebrows. Most of these colored inks are known to contain iron or titanium oxide pigment, which can darken on pulsed or Q-switched laser irradiation (Figs. 5-6 and 5-7). Because a gray tattoo line around the mouth looks infinitely worse than a rust one, it is important to weigh alternative treatment options carefully if darkening is noted.

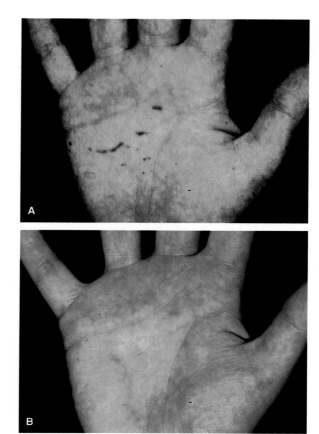

Figure 5-5

Traumatic tattoos resulting from a chemistry explosion involving silver nitrate before (*A*) and 1 month after (*B*) sixth Q-switched alexandrite laser treatment (755 nm, 50 to 100 ns, 3-mm spot size, average fluence, 6.75 J/cm^2).

How old is the tattoo?

Tattoos that have the advantage of age are easier to remove because the body has already broken down and cleared some of the offending pigment. For this reason, older tattoos may require fewer laser treatments than new, multicolored tattoos with greater pigment burden. In addition, newer tattoos have the added disadvantage (in terms of treatment) of containing organometallic dyes in a wide variety of mixed colors that are harder to remove and that have been placed deeply and densely in the dermis. These factors compound the difficulty of treating these tattoos.

Did the patient ever have an allergic or other reaction to the tattoo?

Local allergic and granulomatous reactions have occurred in patients with multicolored tattoos, typically to yellow (cadmium), red (mercury), blue (cobalt), and green (cadmium) inks. Rarely, a systemic allergic reaction can occur. Patients with prior allergic reactions could potentially have a relapse on laser-induced release

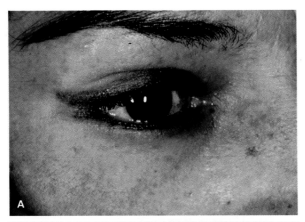

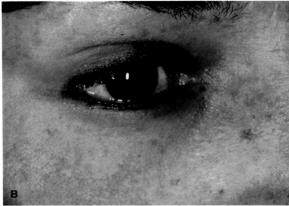

Figure 5-6
Cosmetic eyeliner tattoo before (*A*) and 1 month after (*B*) three treatments using a Q-switched alexandrite laser (755 nm, 50 to 100 ns, 3-mm spot size, average fluence 6 J/cm^2). (A test spot was first placed to exclude the presence of iron or titanium oxide-containing pigment.)

of pigment antigens. Premedication with diphenhydramine (Benadryl), and emergency anaphylactic precautions should be taken in these patients.

Has the patient received any previous treatment to the tattoo?

Many patients have received prior treatment, usually with older modalities such as dermabrasion, excision, cryotherapy, or salabrasion. These treatments may have been slightly effective in removing some tattoo ink, but more than likely, they produced a significant amount of fibrosis and scar as well. Scarring can potentially impede the ability of the laser to remove as much tattoo pigment as it might otherwise be able to clear.

What is the patient's skin type?

Darker skin tones pose a problem for treatment simply because each of the tattoo-specific lasers are also pigment specific. Thus, a certain amount of epidermal pigment usually is sacrificed with tattoo laser treatment. This is more of a cosmetic consideration in patients with darker skin phototypes in terms of the white spots

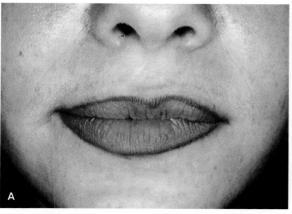

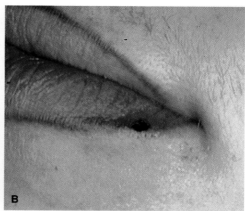

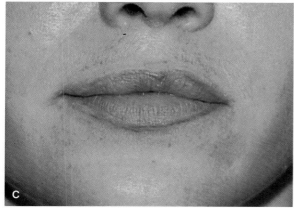

Figure 5-7

Cosmetic lipliner tattoo before (*A*) and after (*B*) a single 3-mm test spot size using a Q-switched alexandrite laser at 6 J/cm^2 showed an immediate blackening response. (*C*) Further treatment was delivered with a high-energy, pulsed CO_2 laser at 500-mJ/pulse energy, 7-watt power, and 10 to 12 laser passes at the vermilion border to achieve virtual tattoo elimination at 1 month. Residual tattoo ink was still visible at the end of the laser resurfacing procedure.

that, while transient in most cases, can persist for several months. In addition, the effectiveness of the laser treatment may be reduced when an excess competing chromophore (eg, melanin) is present. That does not mean that darker skin tones cannot be treated, but additional laser treatments may be necessary, or additional time may be needed between each treatment to allow for ample dermal healing and epidermal repigmentation.

Does the patient have realistic expectations of the proposed treatment?

Patients who think that taking their tattoo off will be as easy as putting it on are fooling themselves and are obviously poor treatment candidates. Patients need to have realistic expectations of the number of treatments that will be needed, and they must be prepared for the discomfort associated with the treatment, the healing time after each session, and the possibility that the tattoo (especially if cosmetic) could actually worsen or be incompletely eliminated.

► **Laser Treatment Protocol**

On establishment of the suitability of a tattoo for treatment, the patient should receive proper preoperative instruction (see Chap. 2). A checklist can help in this process. Once adequately prepared, the patient will also need to sign an informed consent.

In general, tattoo laser treatments are delivered every 4 to 8 weeks to allow for adequate clearing of tattoo fragments and cellular debris and to allow time for proper dermal healing between treatments regardless of the laser system used. The number of treatments required by any one of the Q-switched laser systems to achieve tattoo clearing is essentially the same when using the most updated laser models. Fewer laser treatments are needed with the green-light pulsed dye (510 nm) and frequency-doubled Nd:YAG (532 nm) lasers to clear red and yellow tattoo pigment (Table 5-3). The differences between the lasers lie in the energies used, the number of pulses delivered, and the immediate tissue response on laser impact.

QS Ruby (694 nm)

Fluences ranging 6 to 8 J/cm^2 are used with pulse durations of 25 ns and spot sizes of 5 to 6.5 mm. Immediate tattoo whitening without skin perforation is observed on laser impact. If tissue splatter occurs, the fluence should be adjusted to a lower level.

QS Alexandrite (755 nm)

Average energies of 6 to 7 J/cm^2 with a 3-mm spot size are used for treatment. Initial treatment fluence is determined by individual tissue response. The highest fluence that produces tissue whitening without blood or epidermal splatter is appropriate. Typically, a good starting point is 6 J/cm^2. At this fluence, only the most densely pigmented tattoos produce bleeding (due to conduction of heat to surrounding vessels). If bleeding occurs, the fluence should be reduced in increments of 0.25 J/cm^2 until only tissue whitening is produced. Subsequent treat-

(text continues on page 79)

TABLE 5-3. **CLINICAL TATTOO CLEARANCE**

Tattoo Type	Number of Laser Treatments
Professional	6–12
Amateur	2–6
Cosmetic	1–4
Traumatic	2–6
Medicinal	2–6

LASER TREATMENT OF TATTOOS: PREOPERATIVE CHECKLIST

Type of tattoo:

_____ professional

_____ amateur

_____ traumatic

_____ cosmetic

_____ medicinal

Location of tattoo:

_____ scalp	_____ arms	_____ back
_____ face	_____ legs	_____ abdomen
_____ neck	_____ hands	_____ buttocks
_____ chest	_____ feet	_____ other (_____)

Age of tattoo: _____

Colors present within tattoo:

_____ black	_____ blue	_____ green
_____ red	_____ orange	_____ yellow
_____ violet	_____ tan	_____ brown

Prior treatments (list with dates): _____

Medical problems (list): _____

Allergies: _____

Current medications: _____

Instruction sheet given to patient and thoroughly reviewed _____ (initials/date)

Preoperative photographs taken _____ (initials/date)

Laser treatment scheduled (type/date) _____

Postoperative skin care reviewed and written instructions given to
patient _____ (initials/date)

LASER TREATMENT OF TATTOOS: INFORMED CONSENT

I, _____, understand that I have a tattoo. Dr. _____ has explained to me that although laser surgery is effective in most cases, no guarantees can be made that I will benefit from treatment. I understand that several treatment sessions may be needed to obtain the desired level of improvement. Sometimes, a tattoo will not completely clear but will become lighter; rarely, a tattoo may even worsen after laser treatment.

The most common side effects and complications of this laser treatment are as follows:

1. *Pain.* The snapping and burning sensation of each laser pulse may produce a minimal to moderate amount of discomfort. An anesthetic cream or injection may be used to block the pain if desired.
2. *Bruising.* Immediately after the laser treatment, the area will appear gray or blue-black. The discoloration will fade during the next 7 to 10 days.
3. *Swelling.* Areas most likely to swell are the eyes, hands, and feet. The swelling subsides within 3 to 5 days with regular ice application.
4. *Blisters or scabs.* These usually develop within the first 2 days of treatment and resolve in 1 to 2 weeks.
5. *Skin darkening (hyperpigmentation).* This can occur in the treated areas and will fade within 2 to 6 months. This reaction is more common in patients with olive or dark skin tones and can worsen if the laser-treated area is exposed to the sun.
6. *Skin lightening (hypopigmentation).* This can occur in an area of skin that has already received several treatments. The light spots usually darken or repigment in 3 to 6 months but can be permanent in rare cases.
7. *Scarring.* This is extremely rare but may occur on disruption of the skin's surface. Strict adherence to all advised postoperative instructions will reduce the possibility of this occurrence.
8. *Lesion persistence or worsening.* Some tattoos may not go away completely or may worsen despite the best efforts made by the doctor.
9. *Allergic reaction.* Rarely, an allergic reaction to the release of tattoo pigment in the skin after laser treatment can occur. An allergy to the topical antibiotic ointment may also be possible.

By providing my signature below, I acknowledge that I have read and understood all of the information written above and feel that I have been adequately informed of my alternative treatment options, the risks of the proposed laser surgery, and the risks of not treating my condition. I hereby freely consent to the laser surgery to be performed by Dr. _____ and authorize the taking of clinical photographs, which will be used solely for my medical records unless my physician deems that their anonymous use (in lectures or scientific publications) could benefit medical research and education. They will not be used for advertising without my written permission.

_____   _____
Patient's or Guardian's Signature   Date   Witness' Signature   Date

LASER TREATMENT OF TATTOOS: TREATMENT LOG

Patient name: _____ Age: _____

Skin type: _____

Tattoo type:

_____Professional

_____Amateur

_____Cosmetic

_____Traumatic

_____Medicinal

Previous treatment(s): _____

Treatment #_____   Photos taken: yes/no

Laser used: _____

Fluence or power: _____ (J/cm^2 or watts)

Spot size: _____

Anesthesia: _____

Location treated: _____

Area (in cm) treated: _____

Number of laser pulses: _____

Total treatment time: _____

Skin appearance S/P rx: _____

Complications: _____

Bacitracin/Telfa pad/Tegederm applied: yes/no

Return appointment scheduled: _____ (date)

Home care: bacitracin/Telfa pad/acetaminophen (circle)

LASER TREATMENT OF TATTOOS: SAMPLE OPERATIVE REPORT

Patient name: _____

Diagnosis: _____

Date of operation: _____

Surgeon: _____

Procedure performed: Treatment of (professional/amateur/cosmetic/traumatic)

    tattoo of the _____ [location] with

    the _____ [type] laser

Anesthesia: _____

Total anesthesia time: _____

Laser Procedure

    The patient was brought into the operating room and placed in a supine position. Protective goggles were placed on the patient, and hair-bearing areas were protected. The _____ laser was calibrated to _____ [energy] J/cm^2, and the tattoo on the _____ [location] was treated with a _____-mm spot size. Total area treated was _____ cm. The laser-irradiated area showed the expected whitening response. The patient tolerated the procedure well.

Total operative time: _____

Postoperative wound dressings: Bacitracin ointment, Telfa pad, Tegederm

Postoperative medications: Acetaminophen _____ mg orally every 4 to
    6 hours as needed

Postoperative disposition of patient: Stable and ambulatory

Follow-up appointment scheduled: 1 to 2 months

_____
Surgeon's signature   Date

ments are delivered with the same or slightly increased fluences as determined by the immediate response to laser impact and the tattoo's clinical response to the preceding treatment.

QS Nd:YAG (1064 nm)

Energies ranging from 5 to 6 J/cm^2 are typically used with the largest available (3-mm) spot size. The larger spot size decreases the amount of tissue splatter that had been a common problem with the former use of 1- to 2-mm spots. In addition, lower fluences can be used to achieve the desired clinical response without the risk of textural and pigmentary change that occurred at higher fluences. At times, it may still be necessary to take extra precautions and use Tegaderm or a plastic wrap over the skin during Nd:YAG laser treatment to reduce occupational exposure due to production of tissue debris and blood.

Pulsed Dye (510 nm)

Red, yellow, and orange tattoos can be removed by the 510-nm pulsed dye laser within two to four treatment sessions. An immediate tissue whitening is noted when fluences averaging 3 J/cm^2 are used with a 5-mm spot size. The tattoo can be retreated monthly.

Frequency-Doubled Nd:YAG (532 nm)

Fluences ranging 2 to 3 J/cm^2 using a 3-mm spot size can remove red and sometimes yellow tattoo inks within a few treatment sessions. The treated tattoo turns the desired white color immediately after laser irradiation.

A checklist and laser treatment log can help document all pertinent laser parameters at each treatment session. Operative reports are preferred by many, although they are seldom needed for insurance reimbursement purposes.

▶ Summary

Although more than one laser type remains necessary to remove adequately the different colored inks contained in many professional tattoos, available laser technology has leveled the playing field, and the three Q-switched laser systems (ruby, alexandrite, and Nd:YAG) can all achieve clinically equivalent results within the same number of treatments with similar risk profiles. Similarly, the green-light lasers (510-nm pulsed dye and 532-nm frequency-doubled Nd:YAG) can effectively and equivalently eliminate red tattoo pigment. Removal of green tattoo ink with the Nd:YAG remains a unique problem that can only be remedied with the additional use of a second laser.

Cosmetic tattoos, which are now in fashion, must be approached cautiously because of the presence of iron or titanium oxide–containing pigments. These pigments may turn black on Q-switched or pulsed laser irradiation. Further research is necessary to optimize laser technology and treatment parameters, so that fewer laser sessions are necessary to eliminate a tattoo. Research is also needed to provide further understanding of the obvious chemical reactions that occur on laser impact of tattoo pigment, so that even iron oxide pigments can be eradicated.

Manual of Cutaneous Laser Techniques, by Tina S. Alster.
Lippincott–Raven Publishers, Philadelphia © 1997.

CHAPTER **6**

LASER TREATMENT OF SCARS AND STRIAE

Scar Categorization ▶ *Preoperative Patient Evaluation*
▶ *Laser Treatment Protocol*

Scars and striae have traditionally been difficult lesions to eradicate. The millions of people affected by them have had little in the way of viable treatment options from which to choose until the past few years. Before the discovery that certain lasers could be used to treat scars and striae safely and effectively, treatments such as invasive surgical excisions and grafting procedures, dermabrasion, corticosteroid injections, and radiation therapy were used with varying degrees of success. Unfortunately, most of these treatments often were of little benefit or had side effects that were nearly as severe as the original scar.

In the late 1980s, I began using a vascular-specific pulsed dye laser on hypertrophic scars in port-wine stain patients. It was clear from the beginning that the 585-nm laser could affect more than its intended vascular target because the treated scars became more pliable, less raised and red, and less pruritic. These clinical observations were later substantiated by skin surface textural analyses, erythema spectrometry readings, scar height measurements, and pliability scores, all showing significant improvement within one or two laser sessions. Histopathologic examination of laser-irradiated scars confirmed the suspected improvement in dermal collagen (more fine and fibrillar after laser treatment). They also pointed to a possible etiologic explanation for the laser's effectiveness because regional mast cell numbers were increased in the irradiated scars. Histamine has been shown to both positively and negatively affect collagen synthesis, and its role in laser-induced scar improvement has yet to be determined. Similarly, and perhaps not surprisingly, striae have also shown improvement after 585-nm pulsed dye laser treatment. The fact that striae often demonstrate scar-like features, with early erythema and late fibrosis, could account for the significant improvement seen in some cases.

The introduction of high-energy, pulsed and scanned CO_2 laser technology has enabled cutaneous surgeons to reconsider their treatment of atrophic scars. Atrophic scars have been sanded, dermabraded, peeled, excised, and grafted, but none of these treatments can compare with the vaporizing and tissue-tightening effects achieved through cutaneous laser resurfacing. In addition to removing successive layers of skin, these lasers have shown a unique ability to achieve collagen shrinkage, which clinically enhances the collagen-remodeling process.

Because laser technology is expanding so rapidly and its use in the clinical arena continues to evolve, the range of treatment options for scars may prove confusing. To determine which laser system or combination of laser systems is best for a particular scar, it is imperative to identify properly the type of scar present.

► Scar Categorization

I prefer to group scars based primarily on their clinical features because their distinguishing histologic features described in textbooks often overlap (Table 6-1). In addition, due to the difficulty in quantifying and qualifying collagen on routine light microscopy, histologic differentiation of various scars remains difficult.

Erythematous Scars

Erythematous scars are pink or red and follow the original line of trauma. All scars are typically erythematous in the early phase of wound repair, as an increased number of blood vessels are necessary for the growth of collagen-producing fibro-

TABLE 6-1. CATEGORIZATION OF SCARS

Scar Type	Clinical Features	Histologic Features
Erythematous	Color: pink to red Texture: shiny, few skin markings Morphology: flat	Dilated and increased number of blood vessels; variable fibrosis
Pigmented	Color: tan to brown Texture: shiny, few markings Morphology: flat	Increased melanin at D-E junction; variable fibrosis
Hypertrophic	Color: white, pink, or red Texture: shiny, minimal skin markings Morphology: raised, firm, within wound borders	Thick collagen fibers; scanty mucoid matrix
Keloid	Color: deep red or purple Texture: shiny, minimal to no markings Morphology: raised, firm, extend beyond wound barriers	Thick hyalinized collagen; mucoid matrix; nodular configuration; disorganized arrangement
Atrophic	Color: white or pink Texture: shiny, wrinkled, few markings Morphology: indented or pitted	Thinned epidermis; variable dermal fibrosis

blasts. The presence of erythema beyond 12 months indicates permanence. This is most likely due to a prolongation of angiogenesis and slowed capillary regression during granulation tissue formation. The reason for this occurrence is unclear, but histologic examination of prolonged erythematous scars reveals a larger number of entrapped blood vessels within the newly formed collagen.

Pigmented Scars

Pigmented scars are typically seen in patients with olive or brown skin tones and are probably a result of melanogenesis stimulation by integumental injury. Postinflammatory hyperpigmentation after injury to the dermal–epidermal junction, with displacement of pigment in the dermis, may also account for the pigmentation seen in these scars. With advancing time, the pigmentation usually fades, but some scars remain permanently pigmented.

Hypertrophic Scars

Hypertrophic scars usually develop within the first month after surgery or truma. They can be located on any body area, but the presternal, upper back, and deltoid areas are particularly prone to their development. They appear as pink, firm, raised bands within the boundaries of the inciting wound. The prevalence of collagen synthesis and limited collagen lysis during the remodeling phase of wound repair is the probable cause for their formation. Some hypertrophic scars are symptomatic. Approximately one third of my patients report pruritus or dysesthesia (usually a burning sensation) that is limited to the scars and typically worsens in the evening.

Keloids

Keloids appear as red or purple, raised, firm nodules that, unlike hypertrophic scars, grow beyond the margins of the original sites of injury. They tend to be more invasive of the surrounding normal skin clinically and histologically, with prolongation of the proliferative phase of wound repair and have been described as ''incomplete tumors.'' Although no area of the body is immune to their development, they are commonly seen on the earlobes, shoulders, chest, upper back, and posterior neck. These scars tend to occur with greater frequency in patients with darker skin tones, but any patient can develop this exuberant clinical response. Histologic examination typically shows thick bundles of hyalinized collagen arranged in dense swirls or nodules. Despite these characteristic changes, the fine distinction between a hypertrophic scar and keloid is sometimes best made on clinical grounds alone. I have performed biopsies on numerous hypertrophic or keloid scars that were impossible to categorize both histologically and clinically. Thus, a subset of scars defies categorization. Fortunately, they can still be effectively treated, and my approach to the treatment of hypertrophic scars and keloids is similar (see next section).

Atrophic Scars

Atrophic scars manifest clinically as indented or pitted areas that are limited to previous areas of trauma, surgery, or inflammation. They are particularly common after repeated episodes of inflammatory or cystic acne and are usually seen on the face, anterior chest, shoulders, and upper back. Atrophic scars are typically erythematous early in their development but subsequently fade to hypopigmented or white fibrotic marks.

Striae

Striae appear as linear bands of wrinkled skin that initially appear erythematous and, later, hypopigmented. They typically occur in areas that have undergone excessive stretch, such as the abdomen, hips, and around joints (eg, knees, shoulders) as a result of pregnancy or pubescent growth spurts. The role of hormones, particularly estrogen, in their development has not been fully elucidated, but hormones appear to have an impact. Early striae are clinically and histologically similar to early scars, showing fibrosis and erythema. Late striae, similar to older scars, are clinically hypopigmented and fibrotic. The clinical and histologic similarities of striae to scars may account for their similar responses to pulsed dye laser treatment.

▶ Preoperative Patient Evaluation

Patients with scars who desire laser treatment should be further evaluated to assess whether their particular scars, skin types, and expectations are within a range amenable to treatment. The following questions should be addressed on their initial evaluation.

What type of scar is present?

The type of scar present (erythematous, pigmented, atrophic, keloid, hypertrophic) determines which laser or lasers are indicated for treatment. Proper categorization of the scar also permits correct disclosure of information relevant to the laser chosen, including the number of treatments needed and the anticipated response to each treatment.

How long has the scar or stria been present? If a scar, when did it first appear after surgery or trauma?

Older scars and striae tend to be less erythematous, so an early lesion (less than 1 year old) that presents for treatment may not necessitate laser intervention, especially if it is simply erythematous. When hypertrophy is evident within a scar, however, early intervention has been shown to be helpful in promoting early clinical improvement and decreasing the risk of further worsening. Hypertrophic scars and keloids tend to exhibit initial growth within the first month after surgery or trauma.

Has the scar or stria received prior treatment?

Many patients have received prior treatments to their scars or striae, usually without apparent or significant improvement. Scars that have been treated with cryosurgery, excision, and electrocautery are usually more fibrotic in nature and thus more difficult to treat. Patients should be prepared for the possibility of additional treatments in these circumstances. In contrast, patients who have had silicone or corticosteroid treatment for their scars or striae can undergo laser surgery with the usual and customary tissue response.

Is the scar or stria symptomatic?

Many scars and striae may be pruritic or dysesthetic. Patients frequently report that they require the use of an oral antihistamine at bedtime to reduce the degree of pruritus so that they are able to sleep. Most report that these unpleasant symptoms worsen as the lesions become more raised or red (usually within the first month after injury or trauma).

Are there other, similar lesions present?

Patients who tend to form keloids usually show evidence of other similar scars (check the knees, elbows, and hands). These patients may not be good candidates for cutaneous laser resurfacing because of the risk of new keloid formation, but they can be treated with 585-nm pulsed dye laser without risk of the scar worsening.

What is the patient's skin type?

Patients with darker skin tones (phototypes IV and greater) have a greater amount of epidermal melanin competing for the 585-nm laser light, thereby reducing the amount of energy effectively delivered to dermal scar tissue. This is most important in the treatment of hypertrophic scars and keloids, when the 585-nm pulsed dye laser is used. On the other hand, the obvious problem with performing CO_2 laser resurfacing on deeply pigmented skin is the initial loss of pigment on deepithelialization. Although repigmentation is expected during the first few weeks after cutaneous resurfacing (from the adjacent unlased skin and appendage structures), patients should be forewarned of the definite initial loss of pigment and of the possibility of hyperpigmentation occurring during the repigmentation process.

Has the patient ever been treated with isotretinoin?

Because isotretinoin has been reported to cause hypertrophic scars in patients who have had dermabrasion, it has become routine practice to wait at least 6 to 12 months after completion of a course of isotretinoin before performing a laser resurfacing procedure. The reason for the excessive scarring response is related in some way to isotretinoin's effect on collagen metabolism and wound healing, but the exact mechanism remains unknown.

What does the patient hope to achieve with laser treatment?

Patients who expect their scars to be indistinguishable from normal skin after laser treatment (initial healing notwithstanding) will be disappointed with their results, regardless of any obvious clinical improvement. Scars usually can be improved when the correct laser parameters for the scar type in consideration are used; however, scars can rarely be "erased." Thus, patients should have a clear understanding of the degree of improvement expected for their particular scar categories. I rarely relate my true success rates (average clinical improvement of 80%) to patients. Most patients are happy to hear that a 50% improvement can be expected, as long as the side effect profile is minimal. Patients with symptomatic scars may find relief in the fact that most experience significant improvement, with decreased pruritus and dysesthesia typical after one or two pulsed dye laser treatments.

The use of a checklist during the initial evaluation of a patient can be helpful and should remain a part of the patient's medical record. Once a patient has been determined to be a suitable candidate for laser treatment, baseline preoperative photographs and informed consent should be obtained. Treatment can then proceed using another checklist and treatment log as guides and documentation.

Lᴀꜱᴇʀ ᴛʀᴇᴀᴛᴍᴇɴᴛ ᴏꜰ ꜱᴄᴀʀꜱ ᴀɴᴅ ꜱᴛʀɪᴀᴇ: ᴏᴘᴇʀᴀᴛɪᴠᴇ ᴄʜᴇᴄᴋʟɪꜱᴛ

▶ 585-nm pulsed dye laser in "ready" mode, calibrated to correct fluence with proper handpiece
▶ Anesthetic cream or makeup completely removed with mild soap and water
▶ Safety goggles or glasses on operating personnel and patient
▶ No flammable substances in operating area
▶ Hair protected with wet gauze or headband
▶ Tissues and ice water available for patient comfort
▶ Hand-held fan to cool patient during treatment
▶ Laser tray: bacitracin, polysporin, or mupirocin (Bactroban) ointment, wet gauze, ice pack, Telfa pad or other wound dressing, cotton swabs
▶ Written postoperative instructions given to patient
▶ Return appointment scheduled

LASER TREATMENT OF SCARS AND STRIAE: PREOPERATIVE CHECKLIST

Type of scar:

_____ erythematous

_____ pigmented

_____ hypertrophic

_____ keloid

_____ atrophic

_____ striae

Color:

_____ white

_____ pink (pale)

_____ pink (medium)

_____ red

_____ purple

_____ tan or brown

Location:

_____ scalp	_____ arms	_____ back
_____ face	_____ legs	_____ abdomen
_____ neck	_____ hands	_____ buttocks
_____ chest	_____ feet	_____ other (_____)

Scar height (in mm): _____

Symptoms:

_____ itch

_____ burn

_____ other (_____)

Scar pliability:

_____ supple

_____ yielding

_____ firm

_____ banding

(continued)

LASER TREATMENT OF SCARS AND STRIAE:
PREOPERATIVE CHECKLIST (Continued)

History of:

  (For scars)   _____ isotretinoin use (dates: _____)

                          _____ surgery (type/date: _____)

                          _____ trauma (type/date: _____)

  (For striae)   _____ hormone use/pregnancy (date: _____)

                          _____ >10-lb weight loss/gain (amount/date: _____)

Prior treatments (list with dates): _____

Medical problems (list): _____

Current medications: _____

Allergies: _____

Instruction sheet given to patient and thoroughly reviewed _____ (initials/date)

Informed consent reviewed and signed _____ (initials/date)

Preoperative photographs obtained _____ (initials/date)

Laser treatment scheduled (type/date) _____

LASER TREATMENT OF SCARS AND STRIAE: INFORMED CONSENT

I, _____, understand that I have a _____.
Dr. _____ has explained to me that although laser surgery is effective in most cases, no guarantees can be made that I will benefit from treatment. I understand that several treatment sessions may be needed to obtain the desired level of improvement. Usually, scars and stretch marks do not disappear completely, but will become less noticeable.

The most common side effects and complications of this laser treatment are as follows:

1. *Pain.* The snapping and burning sensation of each laser pulse may produce a minimal to moderate amount of discomfort. An anesthetic cream or injection may be used to block the pain if desired.
2. *Bruising.* Immediately after the laser treatment, the area may appear gray or blue-black in color. The discoloration will fade during the next 7 to 10 days.
3. *Swelling.* Areas most likely to swell are under the eyes and neck. The swelling subsides within 3 to 5 days with regular ice application.
4. *Blisters or scabs.* These rarely develop and can take 1 to 2 weeks to resolve.
5. *Skin darkening (hyperpigmentation).* This can occur in the treated areas and will fade within 2 to 6 months. This reaction is more common in patients with olive or dark skin tones and can worsen if the laser-treated area is exposed to the sun.
6. *Skin lightening (hypopigmentation).* This can occur in an area of skin that has already received several treatments. The light spots usually darken or repigment in 3 to 6 months, but can be permanent in rare cases.
7. *Scarring.* This is extremely rare after this specific laser therapy, but can occur on disruption of the skin's surface. Close adherence to all advised postoperative instructions will reduce the possibility of this occurrence.
8. *Lesion persistence.* Some scars and striae will not go away completely despite the best efforts made by the doctor.

I further understand that, if left untreated, my scars/striae would not be expected to go away on their own.

By providing my signature below, I acknowledge that I have read and understood all of the information written above and feel that I have been adequately informed of my alternative treatment options, the risks of the proposed laser surgery, and the risks of not treating my condition. I hereby freely consent to the laser surgery to be performed by Dr. _____ and authorize the taking of clinical photographs, which will be used solely for my medical records unless my physician deems that their anonymous use (in lectures or scientific publications) could benefit medical research and education. They will not be used for advertising without my written permission.

_____   _____   _____   _____
Patient's or Guardian's Signature   Date   Witness' Signature   Date

► Laser Treatment Protocol

Determining which laser(s) to use should be straightforward once a scar has been properly categorized (Table 6-2).

Flashlamp-Pumped Pulsed Dye Laser (585 nm)

For erythematous, hypertrophic, and keloid scars, the 585-nm pulsed dye laser is used at average fluences of 6 to 7 J/cm^2 when using the 5- or 7-mm spot size and 4 to 5 J/cm^2 when using a 10-mm spot size (Figs. 6-1 to 6-4). Striae are treated at lower fluences of 3 J/cm^2 (Fig. 6-5). Adjacent, nonoverlapping laser pulses are placed to cover the entire scar or stria. An immediate purpuric tissue response should be produced with a variable amount of reactive hyperemia. Irradiated striae do not typically show purpura because of the low fluences used but rather usually appear mildly pink after treatment. Scars that do not become purpuric after laser irradiation (this may occur with keloids) can receive additional overlapping, or double, laser pulses. The treated scar or stria is evaluated 4 to 8 weeks after irradiation, at which time another laser treatment at the same or slightly higher fluence can be delivered. If hyperpigmented laser spots are present within the treated areas, an additional 2 to 4 weeks is given to allow sufficient time for healing before reassessing for further treatment.

Pulsed Dye Laser (510 nm)

The 510-nm pulsed dye laser is used specifically to lighten hyperpigmented scars. Fluences of 2.5 to 3 J/cm^2 are used with a 5-mm spot size. The scar is treated with adjacent nonoverlapping spots so that an immediate ash-white tissue response is produced. The scar is reevaluated after 4 to 6 weeks to determine whether additional treatment is necessary.

TABLE 6-2. **CLINICAL RESPONSES OF SCARS AND STRIAE TO LASER THERAPY**

Scar Type	Laser Used	Number of Treatments Required
Erythematous	585-nm pulsed dye	1–2
Pigmented	510-nm pulsed dye	1–2
Hypertrophic	585-nm pulsed dye	2–4
Keloid	585-nm pulsed dye	2–6
Atrophic	High-energy, pulsed CO_2	1
Striae	585-nm pulsed dye	1–2

LASER TREATMENT OF SCARS AND STRIAE: TREATMENT LOG

Patient name: _____ Age: _____

Skin type: _____

Diagnosis:_____

Previous treatment(s): _____

Treatment #_____   Photos taken: yes/no

Date: _____

    Laser used: _____

    Fluence or power: _____ (J/cm^2 or watts)

    Spot size: _____

    Anesthesia: _____

    Location treated: _____

    Area (in cm) treated: _____

    Number of laser pulses: _____

    Total treatment time: _____

    Skin appearance S/P rx: _____

    Complications: _____

    Bacitracin/Telfa pad applied: yes/no

    Return appointment scheduled: _____ (date)

    Home care: bacitracin/Telfa pad/acetaminophen (circle)

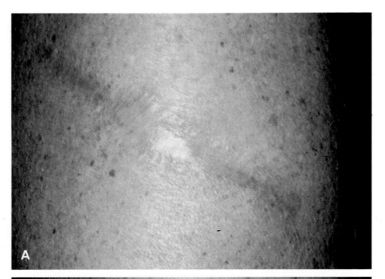

Figure 6-1

(*A*) Erythematous scar with mild hypertrophy on the arm in a 46-year-old woman after surgical excision of a melanoma 2 years earlier. (*B*) Appearance of same scar 2 months after second 585-nm pulsed dye laser treatment (average fluence 4.25 J/cm^2, 10-mm spot size).

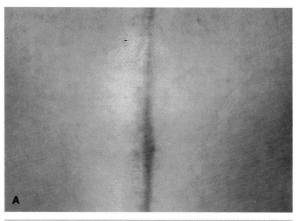

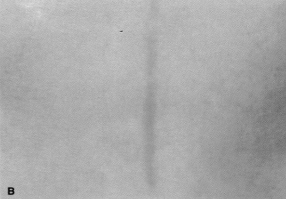

Figure 6-2

Hypertrophic median sternotomy scar in a 4-year-old girl before (*A*) and 2 months after (*B*) second 585-nm pulsed dye laser treatment (average fluence, 6 J/cm^2; 7-mm spot size).

High-Energy Pulsed or Scanned CO$_2$ Laser

Atrophic scars usually resulting from acne, surgery, or trauma can be treated with CO$_2$ laser resurfacing. The entire cosmetic unit should be treated to reduce the possibility of textural or color mismatch. When an isolated scar is present, as can result from surgery or trauma, spot resurfacing can be performed. In either scenario, the scars are deepithelialized across their entire breadth (including the central atrophic portions) to provide an even palette. When large cutaneous areas require resurfacing, this is best accomplished with the use of a scanning handpiece to increase the speed of the procedure. After deepithelialization (within one or two laser passes), a smaller spot size can be used to "sculpt" the shoulders of any remaining individual scars and to even the edges of the cosmetic unit to achieve a clean, finished look (Figs. 6-6 and 6-7).

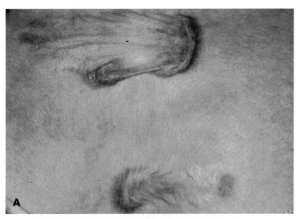

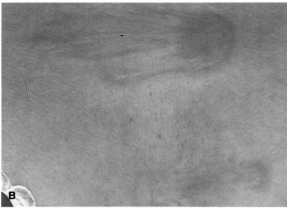

Figure 6-3

(*A*) Keloids on the anterior chest of a 20-year-old woman that occurred after chickenpox as a child. (*B*) Appearance of scars 8 weeks after fourth laser treatment (585-nm pulsed dye laser; average fluence, 6.5 J/cm^2; 7-mm spot).

Laser Resurfacing of Scars: Treatment Pearls

- ▶ Treat entire cosmetic unit or full face (when possible).
- ▶ Treat across the entire scar, then sculpt edges.
- ▶ Do *not* overtreat.
- ▶ Remember to take photographs for documentation.
- ▶ Do not treat if active acneiform lesions are present.
- ▶ Wait at least 6 months after isotretinoin use before resurfacing.

Combined Pulsed CO$_2$ and 585-nm Pulsed Dye Lasers

A combination of high-energy, pulsed CO$_2$ laser scar deepithelialization followed immediately by the 585-nm pulsed dye laser irradiation can be used to treat hypertrophic scars that are not clinically erythematous. The pulsed CO$_2$ system is used,

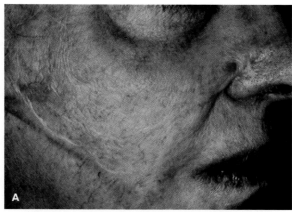

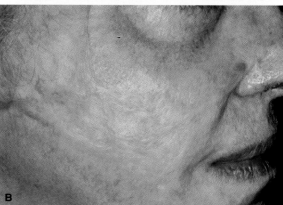

Figure 6-4

(*A*) Hypertrophic burn scars present for 3 years in a 68-year-old woman that were unresponsive to topical steroids, silicone gel, and compression treatments (more than 20 h/day for 2 years). (*B*) Reduction of scar height and erythema and increased pliability observed in scars after third laser treatment (585-nm pulsed dye laser; 7-mm spot size; fluences, 6.25 to 6.75 J/cm²).

not to achieve complete scar vaporization (which leads to scar recurrence), but for deepithelialization purposes only. The addition of 585-nm pulsed dye laser at average fluences of 6 to 6.5 J/cm² using a 7-mm spot size yields an improved clinical result (Fig. 6-8).

The number of laser treatments needed to treat scars is dependent on the type of scar present, the laser used, and each patient's collagen and wound-healing response. In general, more laser sessions are needed to treat hypertrophic and keloid scars to obtain the desired degree of scar flattening and color lightening (see Table 6-2). As mentioned previously, simple vaporization of these hypertrophic scars and keloids produces almost universal scar recurrences and thus should be avoided. Operative reports for these procedures may be necessary for filing insurance claims.

(*text continues on page 103*)

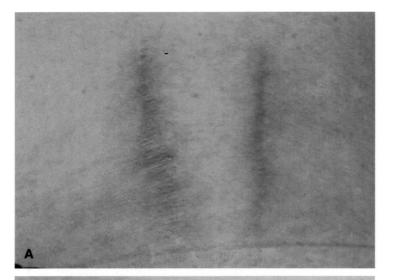

Figure 6-5

Early striae on the abdomen of a 27-year-old woman before (*A*) and 6 weeks after (*B*) a single treatment with the 585-nm pulsed dye laser (3 J/cm^2, 5-mm spot).

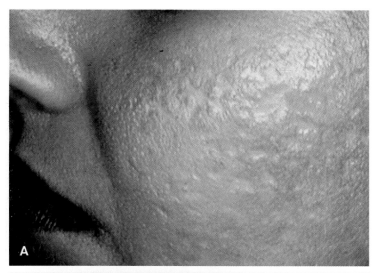

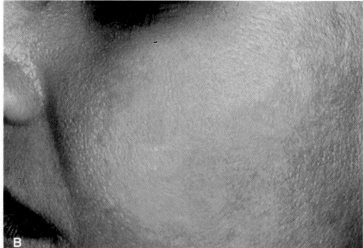

Figure 6-6

Atrophic facial acne scars in a 34-year-old woman before (*A*) and 6 months after (*B*) one treatment using a high-energy, pulsed CO_2 laser (300-mJ energy, 60-watt power, 8-mm square scan, density 6, two passes. Residual scars were further sculpted using a 3-mm spot at 500 mJ/pulse and 7-watt power).

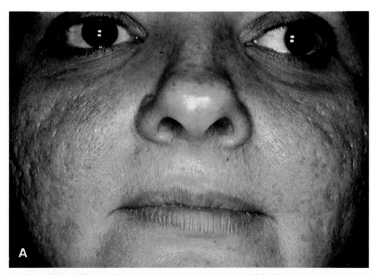

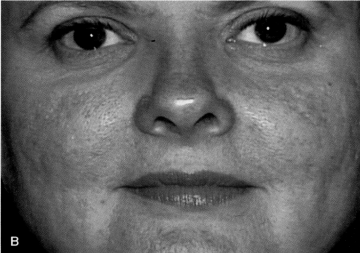

Figure 6-7

Atrophic acne scars before (A) and 6 months after (B) CO_2 laser resurfacing treatment using an 8-mm square scan at 300-mJ energy, 60-watt power, and density of 6. After one pass to deepithelialize and a second pass to achieve collagen shrinkage, individual scars were then treated with one to three additional passes using a 3-mm collimated spot size at 500 mJ/pulse and 7-watt power. Improvement is also seen in infraorbital rhytides and pigmentation.

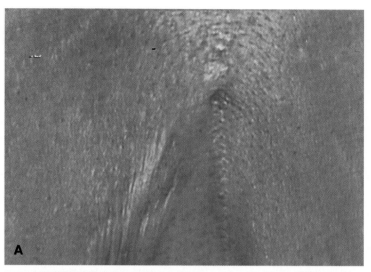

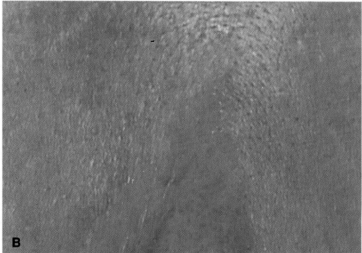

Figure 6-8

Hypopigmented hypertrophic surgical scar of 8 years' duration on the breast of a 50-year-old woman before (A) and 6 months after (B) combined laser treatment using a high-energy pulsed CO_2 laser to deepithelialize the scar (500 mJ/pulse energy, 7-watt power, one or two passes) followed immediately by 585-nm pulsed dye laser irradiation (6.5 J/cm^2, 7-mm spot).

LASER TREATMENT OF HYPERTROPHIC SCARS, KELOIDS, AND STRIAE: SAMPLE OPERATIVE REPORT

Patient name: _____

Diagnosis: _____

Date of operation: _____

Surgeon: _____

Procedure performed: Treatment of _____ [lesion] of

the _____ [location] with the 585-nm flashlamp-pumped

pulsed dye laser

Anesthesia: _____

Total anesthesia time: _____

Laser Procedure

The patient was brought into the operating room and placed in a supine position. Protective goggles were placed on the patient, and hair-bearing areas were protected. The 585-nm pulsed dye laser was calibrated to _____ J/cm^2, and the scar/stria on the _____ [location] was treated with a _____-mm spot size. The laser-irradiated area(s) showed the expected purpuric/erythematous tissue response. The patient tolerated the procedure well.

Total operative time: _____

Postoperative wound dressings: Bacitracin ointment and Telfa pad

Postoperative medications: acetaminophen or a nonsteroidal antiinflammatory medication (eg, ibuprofen) every 4 to 6 hours as needed

Postoperative disposition of patient: Stable and ambulatory

Follow-up appointment scheduled: 6 to 8 weeks

_____
Surgeon's signature   Date

CUTANEOUS LASER RESURFACING OF ATROPHIC SCARS: SAMPLE OPERATIVE REPORT

Patient name: _____

Diagnosis: Atrophic scars

Date of operation: _____

Surgeon: _____

Procedure performed: Laser resurfacing of atrophic scars of

the _____ [location) with a high-energy, pulsed CO_2 laser

Anesthesia: _____

Total anesthesia time: _____

Anesthetist: _____

Laser Procedure

The patient was brought into the operating room and placed in a supine position. Protective eye shields were placed on the patient, and all hair-bearing areas were protected. The involved skin was prepped with Betadine and rinsed thoroughly with water. The high-energy, pulsed CO_2 laser was set to _____ mJ energy and _____ watts power, and the entire _____ [location] was deepithelialized with _____ laser passes. The scar borders were sculpted with _____ laser passes using _____ mJ energy and _____ watts power through a 3-mm handpiece. The laser-irradiated skin surface appeared pink without bleeding.

(continued)

CUTANEOUS LASER RESURFACING OF ATROPHIC SCARS:
SAMPLE OPERATIVE REPORT (Continued)

Total operative time: _____

Postoperative wound dressings

Healing ointments:

   Catrix 10/Theraplex/Aquaphor/Elta/petrolatum

Semiocclusive dressings:

   Vigilon/Flexzan/Second Skin

Postoperative medications:

   Antiviral prophylaxis (eg, acyclovir)

   Antibiotic prophylaxis (eg, azithromycin, ciprofloxacin)

   Pain medication

   Sleeping medication

   Antiinflammatory (eg, acetaminophen, Methylprednisolone, nonsteroidal antiinflammatory)

Postoperative disposition of patient: Stable and ambulatory

Follow-up appointment scheduled: 3 to 4 days

_____
Surgeon's signature   Date

► Summary

Laser technology can now be used to improve different types of scars. It is imperative not only to categorize properly the types of scar present, but also to determine which laser or lasers can best treat them. Because of their high rate of recurrence or worsening, it is not advisable to vaporize scars that are hypertrophic or keloid. When properly used, lasers can achieve superior clinical responses in scar improvement. Future laser technologic advances, as well as the addition of concomitant lasers or other treatments, may eventually yield even better clinical results. By enhancing the remodeling phase of wound healing, abnormal scarring may be prevented. Laser surgery may best be able to accomplish this by triggering regression of blood vessels and, therefore, fibroblasts within the scar. By so doing, further deposition of connective tissue may be halted.

Manual of Cutaneous Laser Techniques, by Tina S. Alster.
Lippincott–Raven Publishers, Philadelphia © 1997.

CHAPTER 7

LASER RESURFACING OF RHYTIDES

CO₂ Resurfacing Lasers ▶ *Rhytide Categorization*
Preoperative Patient Evaluation ▶
Laser Treatment Protocol

In the past few years, the development of pulsed CO_2 lasers has virtually revolutionized the field of cosmetic skin surgery. Prior use of continuous wave (CW) CO_2 lasers to recontour skin yielded excellent clinical results but were limited by excessive heat conduction to the surrounding normal skin. Although these lasers could adequately vaporize tissue, the thermal damage that they caused led to undesirable tissue fibrosis and scar formation. As such, the high risk/benefit ratio of the CW laser procedure prevented its universal acceptance and use.

The new pulsed CO_2 lasers can successfully ablate or vaporize thin layers of skin layer by layer, producing a much narrower zone of cutaneous thermal damage (25 to 70 μm, as compared with 200 to 600 μm with CW systems). As is true with all CO_2 systems, selective absorption of infrared (10,600 nm) light in water-containing tissues such as the epidermis can be achieved. With pulse durations shorter than 1 millisecond, the pulsed CO_2 systems have the advantage of limited penetration (20 μm into skin), confining thermal damage. As a result, sufficient energy is delivered to ablate, rather than burn, tissue.

▶ CO₂ Resurfacing Lasers

Several CO_2 lasers are available for cutaneous resurfacing (Table 7-1). The laser systems that have been used most extensively are the Coherent UltraPulse and Sharplan SilkTouch CO_2 lasers. The UltraPulse laser can produce individual 600-

TABLE 7-1. CO_2 RESURFACING LASERS

Laser Trade Name (Manufacturer)	Laser Specifics
UltraPulse (Coherent)	500 mJ maximum/pulse + computer pattern generator scan 600 μs–1 ms pulse
SilkTouch or FeatherTouch (Sharplan)	Continuous wave flash scanner, <1 ms dwell time 0.2-mm spot in spiral pattern
Surgipulse (Sharplan)	400 mJ maximum/paired pulse 600 μs pulse
TruPulse (Tissue Technologies)	500 mJ maximum/3-mm square spot 60–100 μs pulse, no scan
NovaPulse (Luxar)	Superpulse, 5–8 W 160–900 μs pulse

microsecond to 1-millisecond pulses, with peak energies of 500 mJ. The resultant fluence produced per pulse is greater then the 2- to 5-J/cm^2 ablation threshold of skin. The SilkTouch laser involves the use of a flashscanner attached to a CW CO_2 laser. The flashscanner is a microprocessor-controlled optomechanical device that consists of rotating mirrors resulting in a spiral scan. It can deliver 0.2-mm spots in a spiral pattern so rapidly that the dwell time (or effective pulse duration) on any individual area is less than the 1-millisecond thermal relaxation time of skin. The energy density thus produced by this system is above the ablation threshold of skin.

The Surgipulse laser can achieve maximum energies of 400 mJ delivered in pulse pairs of 600 microseconds each. Although the ablation threshold of skin is reached, less energy actually exceeds it, and less tissue ablation is consequently observed. The TruPulse laser is a 6-watt CO_2 system that produces pulses from 60 to 100 microseconds and pulse energies of more than 5 J/cm^2. The NovaPulse laser is a superpulsed CO_2 system with pulse durations of 160 to 900 microseconds and peak powers of 5 to 8 watts. Unfortunately, superpulsed technology is unable to produce the minimal 2 to 5 J/cm^2 ablation threshold that is critical to achieve tissue vaporization with minimal residual thermal damage. As a result, the risk associated with cutaneous resurfacing is increased.

In addition to the clean layer-by-layer vaporization of skin that these lasers can produce, an immediate skin tightening effect has been observed. This is believed to be due to thermal denaturation of type I collagen, which leads to collagen shrinkage. The combination of tissue ablation and collage shrinkage may account for the extensive collagen remodeling and improvement in surface irregularities observed after laser resurfacing.

Clinical results using these resurfacing lasers have all been impressive. Before determining whether CO_2 laser resurfacing is appropriate for a particular patient, however, it is best to determine the proper categorization of the lesions in question.

TABLE 7-2. **CATEGORIZATION OF RHYTIDES**

Non–Movement-Associated
Perioral
Periorbital
Cheek

Movement-Associated
Forehead
Glabellar
Nasolabial

▶ Categorization of Rhytides

Most facial rhytides result from cumulative photodamage (extrinsic aging) rather than advancing age (intrinsic aging). Ultraviolet light can result in thickening and fragmentation of elastin. Areas most frequently and severely affected by excessive photodamage are the periorbital and perioral regions. Although cigarette smoking can accentuate the development of facial rhytides, particularly perioral lines, by reducing the water content of the skin and rendering it more susceptible to free radicals, its effect is not as significant as cumulative photodamage and genetic predisposition. Patients with pale skin tones show the photodamage most readily. Rhytides can also result from excessive and repetitive muscle movements. Thus, excessive frowning can produce glabellar furrows or "frown lines."

Photoinduced facial rhytides involving the perioral and periorbital regions are particularly responsive to pulsed CO_2 laser treatment and are considered to be primary indications for laser resurfacing (Table 7-2 and Figs. 7-1 to 7-4). On the other hand, rhytides resulting from excessive muscle activity respond less favorably (secondary indications; Figs. 7-5 and 7-6). Even though I have been able to achieve average clinical improvements of greater than 80% even in these latter patients, I do not offer these percentages to prospective patients as an incentive. Patients are willing to accept conservative estimates of anticipated degrees of improvement, especially when the risk profile is minimal.

▶ Preoperative Patient Evaluation

Patients of all ages, skin types, and degrees of photodamage present as possible candidates for cutaneous resurfacing. Because of the prolonged healing phase involved after the procedure, the discomfort associated with the procedure, and the risk of side effects, it is imperative that patients are thoroughly evaluated to determine whether their lesions, skin types, and expectations are conducive to the achievement of optimal results.

Several issues should be addressed to determine the suitability of a patient for cutaneous laser resurfacing (Table 7-3).

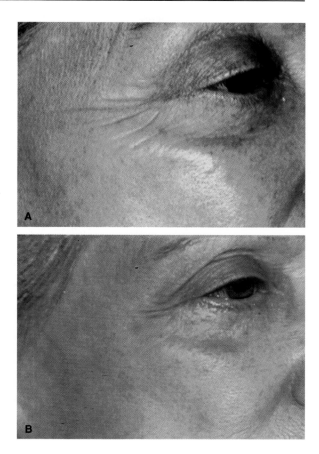

Figure 7-1

Periorbital rhytides in a 70-year-old woman before (*A*) and 6 months after (*B*) CO_2 laser resurfacing (500-mJ/pulse energy, 7-watt power, two laser passes, 3-mm spot).

Does the patient have rhytides that are amenable to laser resurfacing?

Patients with periorbital and perioral rhytides are clearly the best candidates for resurfacing. Movement-associated rhytides involving the glabella and forehead can also be treated but may not show the same degree of improvement. Prominent nasolabial folds can be softened with resurfacing, but jowls are best treated with face-lifting procedures. Similarly, eyelid ptosis and infraorbital fat pads are best treated with blepharoplasty even though laser resurfacing can achieve collagen shrinkage and tissue tightening so that dermatochalasis is significantly improved.

Patients who display more than two distinct regions that are suitable for laser resurfacing should be considered for a full face procedure for the following reasons. First, the intervening cutaneous areas are probably also in need of resurfacing because of the obvious photodamage and probable presence of actinic keratoses and solar lentigines (Fig. 7-7). In addition, it is much easier for the patient to handle the prolonged postoperative erythema when the entire face is treated because camouflaging the Kabuki-mask appearance typically observed after periorbital and perioral resurfacing is difficult.

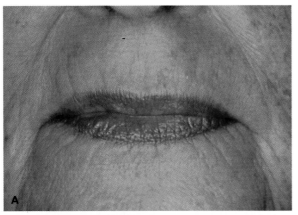

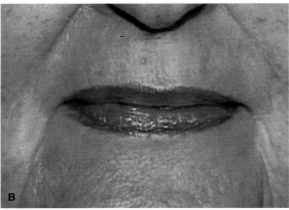

Figure 7-2

Mild perioral rhytides in a 71-year-old woman before (*A*) and 4 months after (*B*) CO_2 laser resurfacing using 500-mJ/pulse energy, 7-watt power, 3-mm spot size, and three laser passes. The nasolabial folds and chin were not treated.

Has the patient received previous treatments for the rhytides?

Patients who have undergone dermabrasions or chemical peels may have developed fibrosis within the treated areas. Fibrotic skin is more dense and thus harder to vaporize. In addition, resurfacing fibrotic skin may unmask underlying peel- or dermabrasion-induced hypopigmentation. Patients who have had blepharoplasties (lower blepharoplasties, in particular) are at greater risk of ectropion formation because of the tissue-tightening effect of laser resurfacing.

Does the patient have other associated cutaneous findings that may also benefit from laser resurfacing?

Patients with enough photodamage to cause the formation of facial rhytides no doubt have other cutaneous lesions that could be treated with laser resurfacing. Solar lentigines and seborrheic and actinic keratoses are commonly seen in these patients, and these lesions are easily cleared with facial resurfacing. Although isolated lentigines are best treated with a pigment-specific laser system (see Chap. 4), the diffuse, scattered variety can often be eliminated in the course of full face resurfacing.

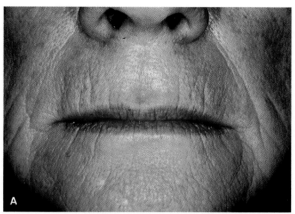

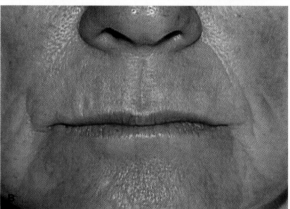

Figure 7-3

(*A*) Moderate perioral rhytides in a 58-year-old woman. (*B*) Appearance 1 year after CO_2 laser resurfacing of perioral, nasolabial, and chin regions using a scanning handpiece at 300-mJ energy, 60-watt power, density 6. Edges of treatment area and vermilion border treated with one additional pass using a 3-mm spot at 500-mJ/pulse energy and 7-watt power.

What is the patient's skin type?

Patients with paler skin tones (phototypes I and II) are the best candidates for laser resurfacing, but any skin type could conceivably be treated. Darker skin tones (especially phototype IV and greater) have a greater tendency to develop postoperative hyperpigmentation. Black-skinned patients should be aware that their skin color will be "wiped away" with laser treatment, but will repigment within the first month after resurfacing.

Has the patient ever experienced cold sores?

Even a remote history of labial herpes is important because reactivation after laser resurfacing is possible. A patient, therefore, who has a history of oral herpes simplex virus who is undergoing perioral laser resurfacing should receive prophylactic antiherpetic medications. Regardless of the history, any patient undergoing full face resurfacing should receive prophylaxis to limit the detrimental effect of reactivation or primary exposure on newly irradiated and granulating skin.

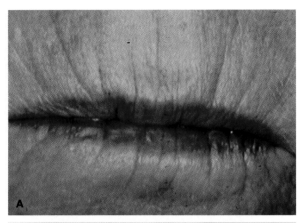

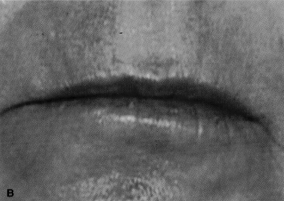

Figure 7-4

(A) Severe perioral rhytides and actinic cheilitis in a 54-year-old woman. (B) Appearance 3 months after CO_2 laser resurfacing of the perioral and lip regions using an 8-mm scanning handpiece at 300-mJ energy, 60-watt power, and density of 6. Vermilion border was treated with an additional two passes using a 3-mm spot at 500-mJ/pulse energy and 7-watt power.

Does the patient have a history of collagen vascular disease or immunologic disorders?

Laser resurfacing entails not only a stressful physical procedure but also a prolonged postoperative course that requires intact immunologic function and collagen repair mechanisms to optimize the healing response. Thus, patients with collagen vascular disorders (eg, scleroderma, lupus erythematosus), autoimmune disorders (eg, vitiligo), or immune deficiencies (eg, human immunodeficiency virus) should be forewarned of the possibility for slower or impaired postoperative healing as well as possible disease reactivation, recurrence, or worsening due to the stress of the procedure.

Does the patient have a tendency to form hypertrophic scars or keloids?

Patients with a scarring tendency are at greater risk for scar formation after cutaneous laser resurfacing, regardless of the laser's specificity and the operator's skill. If the patient is fully aware of the risk, a test area can be lased first to determine whether additional treatment would lead to scarring.

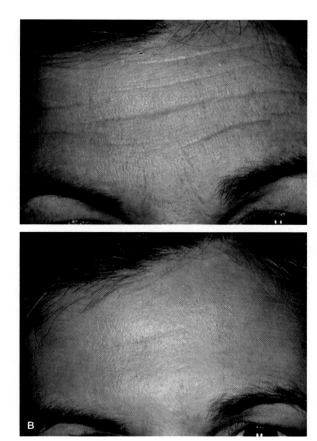

Figure 7-5

Forehead rhytides in a 40-year-old woman before (*A*) and 6 months after (*B*) CO_2 laser resurfacing using an 8-mm scanning handpiece at 300-mJ energy, 60-watt power, density of 6, and two or three laser passes.

Does the patient have realistic expectations of the laser resurfacing procedure?

Patients who expect complete elimination of their rhytides will not be satisfied with laser resurfacing. Certainly, a noticeable improvement is to be expected in all cases, but the actual amount of improvement varies among individual patients and different skin regions. Given the prolonged healing phase that follows laser resurfacing, it is imperative that the patient has a clear understanding of not only the anticipated final clinical result but also the various stages of the procedure and healing process. Patients who are hesitant to accept these side effects are not suitable candidates for treatment.

The use of a checklist when evaluating a patient for cutaneous laser resurfacing is helpful. It can remain in the patient's medical record for reference or be updated at subsequent visits.

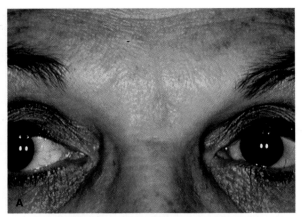

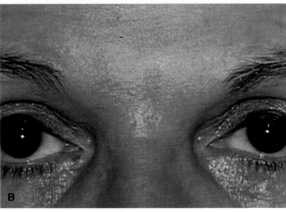

Figure 7-6

A 62-year-old woman with glabellar folds before (*A*) and 6 months after (*B*) CO_2 laser resurfacing using a 5-mm scanning handpiece at 300-mJ energy, 60-watt power, density of 6, and four laser passes.

TABLE 7-3. INDICATIONS FOR CUTANEOUS LASER RESURFACING

Primary Indications	Secondary Indications	Relative Contraindications	Absolute Contraindications
Pale skin types I–II	Dark skin tones (III–IV)	Perpetual UV light exposure	Unrealistic expectations
No UV light exposure	Movement-associated rhytides (glabella/forehead/nasolabial folds)	Prior treatment with skin dyspigmentation or fibrosis	Concomitant isotretinoin use
Non–movement-associated rhytides (perioral/periorbital cheek)	Diffuse facial lentigines	Collagen vascular disease or immune disorder	Concurrent bacterial or viral infection
Actinic cheilitis	Dermal lesions (appendage tumors)	Prior lower blepharoplasty	Presence of ectropion
Epidermal lesions (keratoses)		Tendency to form keloids or hypertrophic scars	

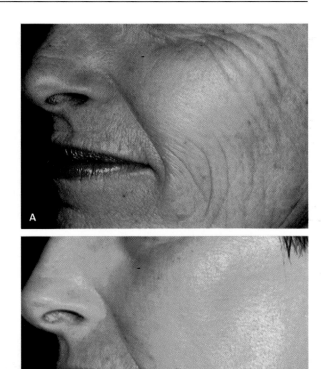

Figure 7-7

(*A*) Prominent cheek rhytides and solar damage in a 59-year-old woman. (*B*) Appearance of skin after full-face CO_2 laser resurfacing using an 8-mm scanning handpiece at 300-mJ energy, 60-watt power, density 6, two or three passes. Skin edges were treated with a 3-mm collimated handpiece at 500-mJ/pulse energy and 7-watt power for a "finished" look.

Once a patient has been determined to be a suitable candidate for treatment, extensive preoperative education is provided (see Chap. 2). Clinical photographs taken before treatment and during the course of healing enable patients to assess their progress. Patients often forget the extent of their conditions before treatment, so it is helpful to have tangible evidence of their preoperative appearance for comparison. Modern technology has facilitated video imaging with computer storage of clinical images that are immediately available for patient viewing (ie, Mirror Image). Thus, expensive and time-consuming film processing is eliminated. In addition, side-by-side clinical images can be generated that are in better alignment than can be achieved by taking free-hand photos. Before undergoing the laser procedure, informed consent must be obtained.

CO_2 LASER RESURFACING: PREOPERATIVE CHECKLIST

Type of rhytides:
_____ periorbital
_____ perioral
_____ nasolabial
_____ glabellar
_____ forehead
_____ cheeks
_____ ears

Severity:
_____ mild
_____ moderate
_____ severe

Associated findings:
_____ upper lid dermatochalasis
_____ lower lid puffiness, bags, hyperpigmentation
_____ jowling
_____ neck laxity

Prior treatments (list with dates): _____

History of:
_____ oral herpes simplex virus
_____ isotretinoin use (last used: _____)
_____ valvular heart disease or bacterial endocarditis
_____ collagen vascular disease (lupus, scleroderma)
_____ immunologic disorder (vitiligo, thyroiditis, anemia)
_____ immunodeficiency

Current medications: _____ _____

Allergies: _____

Instruction sheet given to patient and thoroughly reviewed _____ (initials/date)

Informed consent reviewed and signed _____ (initials/date)

Preoperative photographs obtained _____ (initials/date)

Laser treatment scheduled:
Type _____ Date _____

Postoperative skin care reviewed and written instructions given to patient
_____ (initials/date)

CO₂ LASER RESURFACING: INFORMED CONSENT

Dr. _____ has explained to me that I am a good candidate for laser resurfacing treatment and that although laser surgery has been shown to be highly effective, no guarantees can be made that I will benefit from treatment. I understand that the most common side effects and complications of this laser treatment are the following:

1. *Pain*. The sharp, burning sensation of each laser pulse may produce a moderate to severe amount of discomfort. Anesthetic injections or intravenous sedation will be used to block the pain during the procedure. Oral pain medication will be prescribed for the postoperative period.
2. *Swelling and oozing*. Areas most likely to swell are around the eyes and neck. A clear fluid (serum) will also be present in the lased areas and may create a crust (or scab) if the areas are not kept moist. The swelling, crusting, and oozing stage subsides within 5 to 7 days with regular application of ice and prescribed healing ointments.
3. *Prolonged skin redness*. The laser-treated areas will initially appear bright red in color. After the first week, the redness can be camouflaged with opaque makeup. The redness fades to pink over several weeks, and normal skin color returns in about 3 months.
4. *Skin darkening (hyperpigmentation)*. This can occur in the treated areas and will eventually fade within 2 to 6 months. This reaction is more common in patients with olive or dark skin tones and can worsen if the laser-treated area is exposed to the sun.
5. *Skin lightening (hypopigmentation)*. This can occur in an area of skin that has already received prior treatment or can be a delayed response to the laser surgery. The light spots can darken or repigment in several months, but could be permanent. This is a rare complication.
6. *Scarring*. The risk of this complication is minimal, but it can occur whenever the skin's surface is disrupted. Strict adherence to all advised postoperative instructions will reduce the possibility of this occurrence.
7. *Infection*. A skin infection in the postoperative period can result. This risk in minimized by the use of antibiotics and good skin care.
8. *Allergic reaction*. It is possible that an allergic reaction to an anesthetic, topical cream, or oral medication can occur.
9. *Ectropion*. In rare instances, a downward pull of the eyelids can result after periorbital laser resurfacing.
10. *Acne or milia formation*. Flare-up of acne or formation of milia can occur in the postoperative period.

By providing my signature below, I acknowledge that I have read and understood all of the information written above as well as that contained within the information sheet. I feel that I have been adequately informed of my alternative treatment options, the risks of the proposed laser surgery, and the risks of not treating my condition. I hereby freely consent to the laser surgery to be performed by Dr. _____ and authorize the taking of clinical photographs, which will be used solely for my medical records unless my physician deems that their anonymous use (in lectures or scientific publications) could benefit medical research and education. They will not be used for advertising without my written permission.

_____   _____   _____   _____
Patient's or Guardian's Signature   Date   Witness' Signature   Date

▶ Laser Treatment Protocol

To avoid oversights and to provide adequate procedural documentation, an intra-operative checklist and laser log can be used. Because different cutaneous resurfacing lasers are used at different parameters, what follows are only *suggested* guidelines (Table 7-4). Obviously, the final parameters chosen depend on several factors, including the skin area being treated, the patient's skin type, individual tissue response to treatment, and prior treatments to the area.

In general, all laser treatments are performed by placing adjacent, nonoverlapping spots or patterns over the affected skin area. The skin is wiped with saline or water-soaked gauze between each laser pass to remove any residual, partially desiccated tissue. Additional passes are delivered until the desired clinical endpoint is achieved—usually that of complete lesional effacement in a bloodless and char-free environment.

Thus, the chronology of cutaneous laser resurfacing is as follows:

1. At the time of treatment, the epidermis and a thin portion of the dermis are ablated.
2. A thermal damage zone of 50 to 150 μm persists in the dermis.
3. The laser-induced dermal wound contracts as a result of tissue desiccation and immediate collagen shrinkage.
4. Inflammation cascade begins with collagen remodeling and reepithelialization.

TABLE 7-4. **GENERAL LASER PARAMETERS**

	Periorbital	Perioral	Forehead	Cheeks
UltraPulse				
Energy	250–500 mJ/pulse	300–500 mJ/pulse	300 mJ/60 w/ scan	300 mJ/60 w/ scan
Spot/scan size	3–9 mm	4–9 mm	6–9 mm	6–9 mm
No. of laser passes	1–2	2–4	2	2–3
SilkTouch				
Energy	5–12 W/scan	7.5–20 W/scan	10–20 W/scan	7.5–20 W/scan
Scan size	4–6 mm	4–6 mm	4–6 mm	4–6 mm
No. of laser passes	1–2	2–4	2	2–3
TruPulse				
Energy	350–500 mJ/pulse	500 mJ/pulse	500 mJ/pulse	500 mJ/pulse
Spot size	3 mm	3 mm	3 mm	3 mm
No. of laser passes	2+ "shrink"	2–3+ "shrink"	1–2	2–3+ "shrink"
NovaPulse				
Energy	4–5 W/scan	5–7 W/scan	5–7 W/scan	5–7 W/scan
Scan size	3 mm	3 mm	3 mm	3 mm
No. of laser passes	1–2	2	1–2	2

▽

CO_2 LASER RESURFACING: OPERATIVE CHECKLIST

▶ Resurfacing laser in "ready" mode, calibrated to correct energy with proper handpiece attached

▶ All makeup and other creams completely removed with mild soap and water

▶ Safety goggles or glasses on operating personnel and protective eye shields on patient

▶ No flammable substances in operating area

▶ Hair and body protected with wet gauze and drapes

▶ Laser tray: saline or water-soaked gauze, dry gauze, cotton-tipped applicators, ice water, gloves

▶ Anesthesia setup: injectable lidocaine 1% and 2% with and without epinephrine, syringes, 30-gauge 2.5-inch needles, intravenous tubing and catheters, 500-mL bags of normal saline, intravenous medications (propofol [Diprivan], midazolam [Versed], fentanyl, ketamine, cefazolin [Ancef], promethazine [Phenergan], metoclopramide [Reglan], dexamethasone [Decadron])

▶ Monitoring equipment: electrocardiogram, oxygen saturation and blood pressure monitors

▶ Emergency equipment: defibrillator, oxygen, Ambu bag, oral airway and endotracheal tubes, fire extinguisher

▶ Written postoperative instructions reviewed and given to patient

△

Coherent UltraPulse

The UltraPulse laser can be used with a computer pattern generator (CPG) handpiece, which places 2.25-mm spots in preset patterns at maximum energies of 300 mJ and 60 watts power. Most operators use the hexagonal or square patterns at varying sizes (1 to 9 mm in diameter). Pattern densities can be varied so that spots are placed adjacent to each other, either nonoverlapping (lower density) or overlapping by 10% to 60% (higher density). The 3-mm collimated handpiece is typically used at 350 to 500 mJ/pulse and 3 to 7 watts to treat hard-to-reach areas such as the medial canthal regions, which require more manual dexterity and precise laser spot placement, or at the end of a resurfacing procedure to "sculpt" raised edges of scars or ragged treatment borders (eg, jaw line, scalp line, preauricular area; Figs. 7-8 and 7-9).

CO_2 LASER RESURFACING: TREATMENT LOG

Patient name: _____ Age: _____

Skin type: _____

Diagnosis: _____

Previous treatment(s): _____

Treatment #_____   Photos taken: yes/no

Date: _____

Anesthetist: _____

    Laser used: _____

    Fluence or power: _____ (J/cm^2 or watts)

    Spot or scan size: _____

    Spot or scan pattern: _____

    Location(s) treated: _____

    Total area (in cm) treated: _____

    Total treatment time: _____

    Anesthesia used: _____

    Anesthesia time: _____

    Skin appearance S/P rx: _____

    Complications: _____

    Ointments/wound dressings applied: _____

    Return appointment scheduled: _____ (date)

    Accompanied home by: _____

    Home care: _____

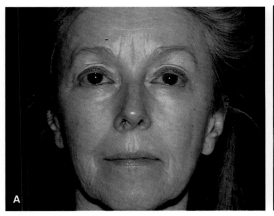
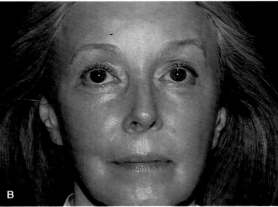

Figure 7-8

Prominent facial rhytides before (A) and 6 weeks after (B) full-face CO_2 laser resurfacing with an 8-mm scanning handpiece at 300-mJ energy, 60-watt power, density of 6, and two or three laser passes. The 3-mm handpiece was used at 500 mJ/pulse and 7 watts to smooth the treatment edges (1 or 2 passes).

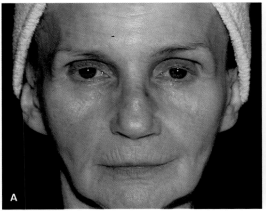
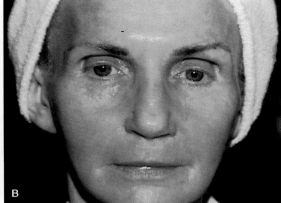

Figure 7-9

A 67-year-old woman before (A) and 2 months after (B) full face CO_2 laser resurfacing using an 8-mm scanning handpiece at 300-mJ energy, 60-watt power, density of 6, and two laser passes.

Sharplan SilkTouch

The SilkTouch flashscanner can be attached to most CO_2 laser systems. The parameters used for resurfacing include spot sizes of 4 to 6 mm and 5- to 20-watt powers. Lower power levels are used for delicate or thin tissue areas such as the periorbital regions. A variable number of laser passes can be delivered to the skin, depending on the the thickness of the skin and the severity of the rhytides. Thicker perioral and cheek skin is typically treated with a greater number of passes than thin periorbital skin.

Tissue Technologies TruPulse

Resurfacing can be performed using the TruPulse with a 3-mm square spot at 500 mJ/pulse energy. When the desired level of tissue ablation has been achieved, a "shrink spatula" is used at 500 mJ/pulse over the desired areas (usually cheeks and perioral regions) to obtain a tightening effect within the skin. Thicker skin areas, such as the perioral and cheek regions, require additional laser passes and the use of the shrink spatula.

Luxar NovaPulse

The NovaPulse laser is used in a superpulsed mode in a repeat exposure pattern for cutaneous resurfacing. The preset programs typically used are A5 (for light ablation) and A14 (for heavy ablation) using a 3-mm scanned handpiece at 4 to 7 watts. These programs correspond to fluences of 60 to 80 mJ/mm^2 delivered to the skin.

Regardless of the laser system chosen for cutaneous resurfacing, there are some basic "dos" and "don'ts" that you should follow (Table 7-5). Because a learning curve exists before meticulous and reproducible results can be obtained, it is imperative that you become as skilled as possible to reduce the potential for complications. Operative reports are essential for proper documentation of the anesthesia used, laser parameters and protocol followed, and postoperative medications prescribed.

TABLE 7-5. CUTANEOUS LASER RESURFACING DO'S AND DON'TS

DO	DON'T
Treat entire cosmetic units	Treat partial cosmetic units
Treat appropriate lesions	Treat anything you are not sure of
Resurface the face	Resurface the neck, chest, or dorsal hands
Treat pale skin tones	Treat tanned skin
Practice laser resurfacing on inanimate objects (eg, fruits, vegetables)	Practice your techniques on patients until you are skilled

CO$_2$ LASER RESURFACING: SAMPLE OPERATIVE REPORT

Patient name: _____

Diagnosis: Severe facial photodamage with rhytides

Date of operation: _____

Patient status: Outpatient

Surgeon: _____

Procedure performed: Resurfacing of facial skin with pulsed CO$_2$ laser

Anesthetist: _____

Anesthesia: _____

Total anesthesia time: _____

Laser Procedure

The patient was brought into the operating room and placed in a supine position. Wet drapes were placed over the patient, and all exposed hair-bearing areas were dampened with water. The facial skin was prepared with a non–alcohol-containing cleanser. Protective nonreflective metal eye shields were placed on the patient.

The pulsed CO$_2$ laser was calibrated to _____ [energy/power] and a _____-mm handpiece was used to treat the _____ [location] in adjacent, nonoverlapping pulses/scans. A total of _____ laser passes were delivered. The skin was wiped with saline-soaked gauze between each pass to remove partially desiccated tissue.

The laser-irradiated skin showed a clean, pale pink hue without bleeding. The patient tolerated the procedure well.

Total procedure time: _____

Total recovery period: _____

Postoperative medications: _____

Postoperative disposition of patient: Stable and ambulatory

Follow-up appointment scheduled: _____ (date)

_____
Surgeon's signature   Date

▶ Summary

Although face-lifts and blepharoplasties remain the treatments of choice for sagging skin, the latest CO_2 laser technology has revolutionized the approach to facial rejuvenation of rhytides. In the past, cutaneous resurfacing had been limited to chemical peels and dermabrasion, which had much higher risk/benefit ratios because of the development of significant pigmentary alterations, fibrosis, and scars. The advantage of the new pulsed and scanned CO_2 laser systems is that the skin can be removed in a controlled and precise layer-by-layer manner until the desired clinical endpoint is reached. Because there is no char or blood, clear visualization of the tissue and its response during treatment is possible, unlike during a dermabrasion or chemical peel. Despite the precise laser parameters and improved visualization of treatment endpoints, complications can still occur with laser resurfacing. Laser technique, clinical experience, and postoperative wound management are all essential elements to ensure successful treatment and reduce the risk of complications.

Certainly, the largest drawback to the laser resurfacing procedure is the prolonged postoperative course, including erythema, which typically persists for 2 months or more. Shorter-pulsed CO_2 lasers and erbium YAG lasers may be at the forefront of the next laser generation as a result of their potential to decrease the amount and duration of postoperative crusting and erythema. Until then, appropriate patient selection and preparation, as well as the use of proper operative technique and postoperative management, can enhance the clinical results obtained, with minimal complications.

Manual of Cutaneous Laser Techniques, by Tina S. Alster.
Lippincott–Raven Publishers, Philadelphia © 1997.

CHAPTER 8

MISCELLANEOUS AND COMBINATION LASER APPLICATIONS

CO_2 Laser Blepharoplasty ► *Laser Hair Transplantation* ► *Laser-Assisted Hair Removal*

► CO_2 Laser Blepharoplasty

Although the CO_2 laser has been used to perform soft tissue surgery for several decades, it was not until 1980 that the first laser blepharoplasty was performed. The technique was virtually ignored until advances in cutaneous laser resurfacing resurrected the CO_2 laser's prominence in aesthetic surgery. Now, upper and lower laser blepharoplasties are becoming more common.

In the hands of an experienced user, there are few disadvantages to using the CO_2 laser for blepharoplasty surgery (Table 8-1). Its advantages are related to its ability to coagulate vessels with diameters less than 1 mm, so that little bleeding is encountered. This, along with the associated reduction in intraoperative time, leads to a quicker recovery period with less swelling and bruising. Disadvantages of laser blepharoplasty tend to be centered around safety issues; flammable surgical drapes, skin preparation solutions, and oxygen could potentially cause an intraoperative fire with inadvertent burns. In addition, scleral or ocular injury can occur if proper eye protection is not enforced. Because of the lack of tactile feedback available to the operator as the laser incises the tissue, the surgeon must develop the ability to recognize visually the depth of dissection. Failure to do so can result in the accidental division of deep structures, including the levator aponeurosis

TABLE 8-1. CO$_2$ LASER BLEPHAROPLASTY

Advantages	Disadvantages
Decreased bleeding	Fire hazards
Shorter intraoperative times	Risk of ocular injury
Quicker recovery period	Technique-dependent results
Reduced postoperative edema and ecchymoses	

and, with inadequate eye protection, the sclera. Thus, safety precautions and operator skill are paramount to the procedure's success.

In summary, the CO$_2$ laser is particularly well suited to performing blepharoplasty surgery. When used as an incisional device, it offers several advantages, including improved hemostasis, decreased intraoperative time, and decreased postoperative edema and ecchymosis. Proper surgical technique and safety measures are essential to the safe and effective use of this device.

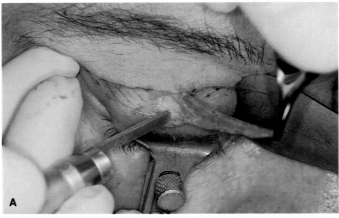

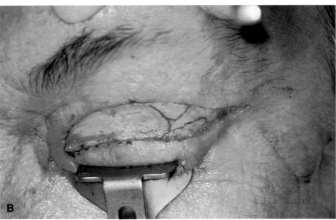

Figure 8-1

Upper laser blepharoplasty in a 45-year-old woman. (*A*) Intraoperative photograph shows elevation of the skin muscle flap. The David-Baker clamp provides protection for the eye. (*B*) The skin muscle flap has been removed. Note the terminal branch of the lacrimal artery on the anterior surface of the orbicularis muscle which has been spared to avoid intraoperative hemorrhage. The patient shown preoperatively (*C*) and 18 days after (*D*) upper eyelid blepharoplasty, transconjunctival lower eyelid blepharoplasty and periorbital CO$_2$ laser resurfacing. (Courtesy of Brian S. Biesman, MD) *(continued)*

Treatment Protocol

Laser blepharoplasty can be performed in an office setting using local anesthesia, intravenous sedation, or both. There are several CO_2 lasers from which to choose. Coherent, Sharplan, Luxar, and Tissue Technologies all manufacture lasers capable of performing incisional surgery and cutaneous resurfacing. The initial incision is made through skin and orbicularis muscle with a 0.1- or 0.2-mm handpiece held perpendicular to the skin at 5 to 6 watts, although settings may vary from laser to laser. The depth of incision is controlled by adjusting the laser power setting, the distance the laser is held from the skin (with more cutting at maximum beam focus), and the speed with which the beam is moved. The orbital septum is opened, and herniating orbital fat is excised. Large vessels visible within the fat can be coagulated with a defocused beam before their division or, preferably, avoided altogether (they bleed if divided and may retract into the orbit, potentially threatening vision). The skin is closed with interrupted, running, or subcuticular sutures (Fig. 8-1).

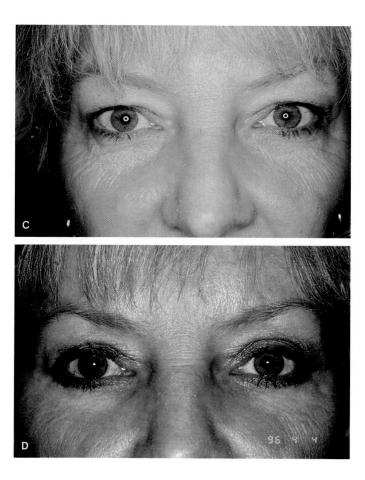

Figure 8-1 *(continued)*

Lower-eyelid blepharoplasty is often performed using a transconjunctival approach, which permits dissection of orbital fat without disruption of the orbital septum. Because division of the orbital septum can produce undesirable scarring within the eyelid, leading to scleral show and lower eyelid retraction, it is best to avoid this approach if possible. The CO_2 laser is used in a cutting mode to divide the conjunctiva and lower eyelid retractors, thereby exposing the orbital fat. The lower eyelid is then retracted inferiorly with a laser-safe retractor, which is used as a surface against which the fat can be transected with the laser. The conjunctival wounds do not require closure. Laser resurfacing may be performed immediately after transconjunctival blepharoplasty, but should be delayed for 3 to 6 months if an external approach is used.

▶ Laser Hair Transplantation

Hair transplantation was initially performed using round punch grafts of hair-bearing skin, which were placed in thinning or balding areas (recipient sites). This technique had distinct disadvantages, including initial hair loss within the recipient site due to removal of residual hair by the application of the punch. In areas of total alopecia, the initial grafts would give the patient an appearance of a Kewpie doll until the intervening areas could be further transplanted. Finally, it was difficult to achieve a natural-appearing hairline with punch grafts alone.

With the introduction of minigrafting, in which smaller grafts containing one to six hairs were transplanted at a time, these disadvantages were markedly diminished. Unfortunately, despite the use of smaller grafts, the "slits" that were made at the recipient sites presented a few drawbacks of their own. First, compression of the grafts within the slits yielded an undesirable appearance of dark lines coursing through the scalp. Second, because fewer hairs were being transplanted at a time, more grafts became necessary. Finally, grafts could be squeezed by the narrow slit, causing an elevation or depression of the skin.

When the slits are made wider (1 to 2 mm), the problems of graft compression and unevenness with slit-grafting are eliminated. This can now be accomplished with the use of a high-energy, pulsed CO_2 laser (older CW CO_2 lasers were associated with unacceptably wide zones of thermal damage at the incision sites). The latest CO_2 laser technology produces such brief pulses of high-energy that thermal damage is limited to 20 to 50 μm in the skin. Thus, normal hair follicles are spared, and bleeding is minimized (Table 8-2).

Hair distribution after laser slit transplantation is significantly more natural-appearing and can yield hair densities comparable to traditional punch grafting. The use of a laser in transplantation can eliminate many of the disadvantages associated with punch and slit grafting, but requires much practice to incorporate yet another technique in what is already a complicated endeavor. Overall, however, it appears that when properly used, laser slit hair transplantation can yield better clinical results and may be associated with few postoperative side effects.

TABLE 8-2. **HAIR TRANSPLANTATION: COMPARISON OF TECHNIQUES**

	Punch Grafts	**Scalpel Slits**	**Laser Slits**
Hair density	Good	Less dense	Good
Hairline	Unnatural	More natural	Most natural
Hemostasis	Poor	Better	Superior
Complications	Poor cosmesis	Graft compression	Laser plume
	Loss of hair in recipient punch sites	Graft elevation and depression	More crusting
			Added technique
Advantages	Fast	Fast	Fewer therapy sessions
	Single technique	Single technique	Faster hair regrowth
			No graft compression
			No graft elevation or depression

Laser Treatment Protocol

Tumescent anesthesia with field blocks is typically used to obtain adequate anesthesia for the procedure. The donor sites are obtained from excised strips of hairy skin at the inferior and superior occipital areas for fine and coarse hairs, respectively. Finer hairs are transplanted at the hairline to achieve a more natural appearance. Typically, 350 to 400 slit grafts and 100 micrografts can be obtained from each donor strip. Laser slits are produced with a 0.2-mm focused spot at 15 watts and 350 to 450-mJ energy, which on tissue contraction, expands the slit to 0.5 mm. The distance between each adjacent slit made in a single session is 3 mm, with 1-mm spacing anteriorly and posteriorly. Using this precisely uneven pattern, laser slit grafting can produce excellent results in three sessions. The last session is conventional nonlaser grafting to limit thermal injury to the skin. A computer-driven laser scanner has been developed that can accurately place the slits in the aforementioned pattern in a fast and consistent fashion. In addition, because of to the hemostatic effect of the laser and its ability to improve tissue visualization during surgery, less postoperative pain and edema have been reported.

▶ Laser-Assisted Hair Removal

The concept of using a laser to target hair follicles to eliminate hair is enticing. Traditional forms of treatment have included waxing, shaving, tweezing or plucking, and electrolysis. Unlike the temporary effect of waxing, plucking, and shaving, electrolysis has been the only form of therapy that could potentially remove hair permanently. But even electrolysis, which involves the insertion of a fine needle into the hair follicle through which an electric current is passed to destroy the hair bulb, has not been uniformly successful. In fact, a success rate of only 30% is typical. The process is tedious, long, and uncomfortable, with several sessions needed to defoliate any section of skin. The effectiveness of electrolysis and its risk of side effects, notably scarring, hypopigmentation, or hyperpigmentation, is based on the skill of the operator and the limitations of using a nonselective technology.

Laser hair removal is a relatively new but promising process. A number of laser companies have worked on developing technology that would involve the delivery of laser light directly to the hair follicle target. Because of the known effect of red and near-infrared light on dermal pigment, the use of ruby (694-nm red light), alexandrite (755 nm red light) and Nd:YAG (1064-nm infrared light) lasers to target hair follicles made sense. Patients with dark hair have a greater potential for success because of the increased amount of pigment present in their hair shafts and follicular papillae. This is particularly true for hairs in anagen. The use of a carbon-based solution to highlight the hair follicle enhances the follicle's visibility and promotes conductivity regardless of the hair color; it also permits the use of lower energies to achieve the same destructive effect. Thus, hair removal would not be dependent on hair color or follicular morphology. This latter concept of using a carbon solution in conjunction with laser treatment to target hair selectively has been patented under the name SoftLight, which is the only laser device with Food and Drug Administration approval for hair removal (as of December 1996). Other investigative laser systems, such as Epilase (Palomar Corporation) and Photogenica (Cynosure), which involve the use of long-pulsed ruby or alexandrite lasers, and other methods (eg, PDT using topical aminolevulinic acid) may also prove successful in permanently removing unwanted hair.

Laser-assisted hair removal is being performed with encouraging results. Its distinct advantage lies in its enhanced selectivity and, thus, effectiveness in permanently eradicating hair or slowing hair regrowth. It is fast and associated with minimal patient discomfort. As more laser systems are approved for use in hair removal, treatment protocols and parameters will be optimized to achieve the best possible outcomes.

Laser Treatment Protocol

The SoftLight hair removal laser (Thermolase Corporation) is actually a low-energy, non–Q-switched Nd:YAG laser. Immediately before laser irradiation, the area to be treated is waxed to remove the hair and to permit the follicular infiltration of the patented carbon-based solution that is massaged into the skin. The black pigment is targeted by the laser, and heat is conducted to the hair papillae, thus destroying the hair at its root (Fig. 8-2). There is an immediate crackling or rapid-fire popping sound that is produced by the laser pulses. The pain experienced is minimal, but the cumulative effect of the laser pulses can generate enough heat to be uncomfortable. More sensitive areas, such as the lip and bikini line, may actually be painful to treat. Whatever is felt during the procedure instantly ceases when the treatment is stopped. The treated area may be pink—usually a result of the waxing procedure, rather than the lasing procedure—but fades within hours (Fig. 8-3).

A single treatment can be expected to result in at least a reduction in hair growth and hair thickness, but the number of treatments required to obtain a cosmetically acceptable result varies among patients and body parts. Clinical experience thus far indicates that the chin is a particularly stubborn or recalcitrant area, possibly because of the thick, coarse nature of the hairs or the rapid growth of these hairs. Hairs in the bikini area at the upper medial thigh and lower abdomen and perineum tend to be more responsive to treatment.

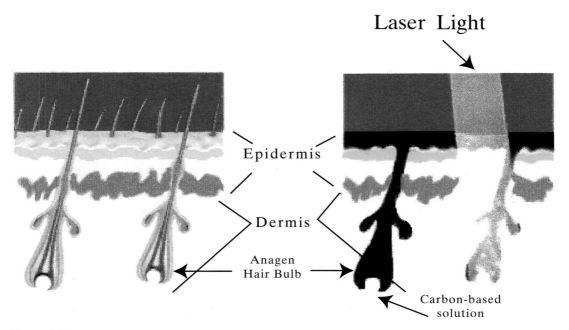

Figure 8-2

Cross section of skin showing carbon-based solution in hair papilla. Laser light targets black pigment.

Treatments are typically delivered at 4- to 16-week intervals, depending on the rate of regrowth, using a 10-mm spot at fluences of 2.5 to 3 J/cm^2. Because the technology is relatively new, the average number of treatments required per area remains unknown, but all patients should be prepared for at least two treatments. At best, the patient can expect an 80% reduction of hairs if all hairs in anagen are eliminated. Some patients find that a single treatment, while not able to eliminate hair completely, can effect a response that is so favorable that they are not inclined to undergo further treatment.

The advantages of laser hair removal over conventional treatments (Fig. 8-4) include an enhanced ability to eradicate hair growth permanently (over 30%), finer texture of hairs seen on regrowth, paler color of hair on regrowth, and slower hair regrowth in general. Obvious disadvantages include the variable responses of individual patients (due to hair texture and location) and the expense. When one compares the laser-assisted hair removal process to other treatments such as waxing and electrolysis, however, it is clear that fewer treatment sessions are necessary in the long-term, and thus, the overall cost may actually be less. Large areas can be treated in one sitting, compared with the slow tedious method of electrolysis, and side effects such as scarring and pigmentary alteration are minimized because of the high selectivity of the laser (Table 8-3).

When first evaluating a patient for laser-assisted hair removal, a checklist should be used to ascertain and document which regions require treatment, whether prior treatments had been tried, and the presence of other medical prob-

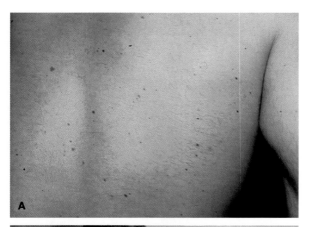

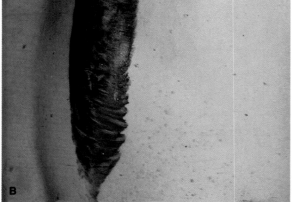

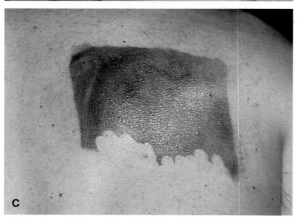

Figure 8-3

(*A*) Terminal hair on the back before treatment. (*B*) Same area after waxing and with application of carbon-based solution. (*C*) Midway through SoftLight treatment showing large footprint of laser spots at bottom field.

ELECTROLYSIS   WAX   SHAVE

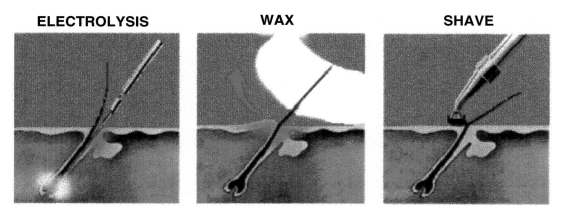

Figure 8-4
Various nonselective hair removal processes.

lems pertinent to the hair growth, such as hormonal imbalance or thyroid disease. If laser hair removal is chosen, an informed consent should be obtained that clearly outlines the risks of the procedure and the fact that more than a single treatment is generally necessary. A treatment checklist and log are helpful to track the number of treatments delivered, locations treated, and parameters used for each treatment.

TABLE 8-3. **COMPARISON OF HAIR REMOVAL TECHNIQUES**

Waxing	Electrolysis	Laser
Lifetime sessions	Multiple sessions	Fewer sessions
Not permanent	About 30% permanent	>30% permanent
Nonselective technique	Technique dependent	Very selective for hair target
Painful	Painful	Less painful
Fast	Slow	Fast
Less expensive	Expensive	Expensive
Large treatment areas	Small treatment areas	Large treatment areas
Few side effects	More side effects	Few side effects

LASER-ASSISTED HAIR REMOVAL: INFORMED CONSENT

I, _____, consent to and authorize Dr. _____ to perform multiple laser-assisted hair removal treatments on me.

The areas to be treated are _____.
The nature and purpose of the laser treatments have been explained to me, and any questions that I have regarding the treatment have been answered to my satisfaction. I understand that it may not be possible to totally eliminate my unwanted hair with the laser treatment.

I understand that the treatment may involve risks of complication or injury from both known and unknown causes, and I freely assume these risks. These risks include, but are not limited to, the following:

1. Skin burns from hot wax, laser treatment, or both
2. Temporary redness in the treated area, which usually lasts for a few hours
3. Swelling in the treated area, which usually subsides within 24 hours
4. Pigmentary (light or dark) changes in the skin from waxing, laser treatment, or both
5. Pain during the procedure and skin tenderness or burning and stinging sensations, which last for 24 hours after the procedure
6. Superficial skin infection
7. Folliculitis from ingrown hairs
8. Allergic reaction to a topical solution or product used on the skin

I certify that I have read this entire Informed Consent and that I understand and agree to the information provided in this form. I have received, reviewed, and understood all information contained in the posttreatment information sheet. I freely and voluntarily consent to the laser-assisted hair removal treatment.

_____   _____
Patient's or Guardian's Signature   Date

_____   _____
Witness' Signature   Date

LASER-ASSISTED HAIR REMOVAL: PREOPERATIVE CHECKLIST

Areas involved:

__ upper lip __ neck __ back __ thighs __ under arms

__ chin __ chest __ shoulders __ lower legs __ upper arms

__ cheeks __ breasts __ buttocks __ feet __ forearms

__ eyebrows __ abdomen __ bikini area __ hands __ other (__)

Prior treatments:

__ electrolysis (body area: _____ dates: _____ last rx: _____)

__ waxing (body area: _____ dates: _____ last rx: _____)

__ laser treatment (body area: ____ dates: _____ last rx: _____)

__ Isotretinoin (Accutane) (dates: _____)

__ Minoxidil (Rogaine) (body area: _____ dates: _____ last rx: _____)

Current method of hair removal: _____

Medical history (eg, hormone inbalance, thyroid disease): _____

Medications: _____

Allergies: _____

LASER-ASSISTED HAIR REMOVAL: TREATMENT CHECKLIST AND LOG

Patient name: _____

Age: _____

Previous treatments: _____

No. Rx	Date	Operator Initials	Area(s) Treated	Wax (+ / −)	Carbon (+ / −)	Lasr Rx (J/cm^2)	Comments
1.							
2.							
3.							
4.							
5.							
6.							
7.							
8.							

Manual of Cutaneous Laser Techniques, by Tina S. Alster.
Lippincott–Raven Publishers, Philadelphia © 1997.

CHAPTER **9**

SKIN CARE AND MAINTENANCE AFTER LASER TREATMENT

After Vascular Lesion Laser Treatment ▶
After Pigmented Lesion and Tattoo Laser Treatment ▶
After CO$_2$ Laser Resurfacing

Laser-treated skin requires special care, regardless of the laser used or the lesion treated. Different laser treatments, however, produce various skin responses and thus require different postoperative regimens.

▶ After Vascular Lesion Laser Treatment

The skin appears purpuric with surrounding tissue hyperemia immediately after 585-nm pulsed dye laser treatment (Fig. 9-1). After quasi-CW laser treatments, such as with copper vapor, krypton, KTP, and argon-pumped dye lasers, the skin appears minimally pink, with a crust forming within a few days. Patients should be instructed to avoid sun exposure and to apply a topical antibiotic ointment to the irradiated areas for the 7- to 10-day healing period typical after treatment with these lasers. A mild, nonirritating soap such as Catrix Correction Cream Wash or Aquanil can be used twice daily on the treated areas.

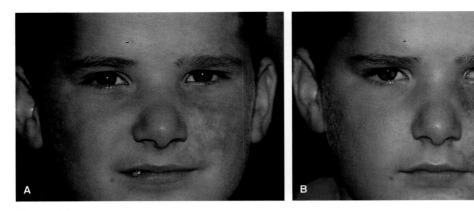

Figure 9-1

A 10-year-old boy with a port-wine stain before (*A*) and immediately after (*B*) 585-nm pulsed dye laser treatment. Laser-induced purpura and surrounding tissue hyperemic response are visible.

► After Pigmented Lesion and Tattoo Laser Treatment

The laser-irradiated areas immediately appear ash-white or purpuric (Fig. 9-2), depending on the amount of pigment present in the lesion. The greater the amount of pigment or tattoo ink present, the greater is the ash-white tissue response. The laser-irradiated skin should be cleansed gently with mild soap and water twice daily during the 1-week healing period. Antibiotic ointment is applied after each cleansing until all areas are healed. The skin is protected from sun exposure during the recovery process and between laser treatments by application of sunscreen and bandages.

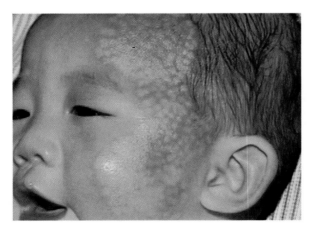

Figure 9-2

Infant with nevus of Ota immediately following QS alexandrite laser treatment. Note ash-white tissue response and no bleeding or epidermal disruption with adjacent 3-mm spots.

INSTRUCTIONS FOR SKIN CARE AFTER LASER TREATMENT FOR VASCULAR LESIONS, LENTIGINES, TATTOOS, HYPERTROPHIC SCARS, OR KELOIDS

The treated area is *extremely delicate* and *must be handled with care* during the initial healing phase (7 to 10 days). It may take a few weeks after the bruising or scabs disappear for fading to occur. Your response to treatment, therefore, will not be evaluated for several weeks, when the healing process is complete.

1. Apply bacitracin, Polysporin, or Bactroban ointment (*not* Neosporin) to the treated area, and cover with a bandage (Telfa pad with adhesive) one to two times a day for 7 to 10 days.
2. Showers are permitted, but prolonged bathing is not advised. Gently pat the area dry with a soft cloth. *Do not rub* with a towel or washcloth because the area is extremely delicate while healing.
3. Any discomfort you feel (usually not lasting more than 6 hours) should be relieved with acetaminophen (Tylenol). *Do not ingest aspirin* or aspirin-containing medicines during the healing phase (1 to 2 weeks).
4. To prevent or reduce swelling, apply an ice pack to the area. The ice should be wrapped in a soft cloth and applied for 10 to 15 minutes each hour for 4 hours.
5. *Do not tan* the laser-treated area. Use a sunscreen with SPF 15 or greater throughout the course of treatment.
6. Avoid swimming and contact sports while the skin is healing.
7. Do not pop any blisters or pick any scabs that develop.

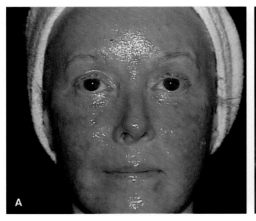 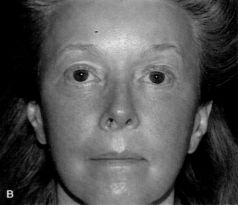

Figure 9-3

(*A*) Patient 4 days after full-face laser resurfacing procedure. There is intense erythema, swelling, and serous discharge, but no crusting or evidence of infection. (*B*) Same patient 4 days later (postoperative day 8) with decreased erythema and swelling and no discharge. She is able to apply camouflage makeup at this time under supervision.

▶ After CO$_2$ Laser Resurfacing

Immediately after cutaneous laser resurfacing, the treated skin appears pale pink and slightly swollen. The erythema and edema intensify during the first 24 to 48 hours (Fig. 9-3). During this critical period, patients should be encouraged to keep the laser-irradiated area moist, either with continuous application of healing ointments such as Catrix-10, Aquaphor, Theraplex, or Elta, or with coverage by hydrogel wound dressings such as Vigilon, Second Skin, or Flexzan (Table 9-1). Application of ice to the treated skin and around-the-clock antiinflammatory medications, such as acetaminophen, help to minimize swelling. In patients in whom large skin areas have been resurfaced or in those who have a history of herpes labialis, a 10-day course of oral antiherpetic medication (eg, acyclovir) is prescribed. Antibiotics can be given intraoperatively, postoperatively, or at both times in patients with a history of valvular heart disease and in those who have had extensive areas of skin treated. The use of topical antibiotics on acutely resurfaced skin is avoided because of a high incidence of allergic and irritative tissue responses.

TABLE 9–1. **CUTANEOUS LASER RESURFACING: POSTOPERATIVE PROTOCOL**

Skin Care
Ice or cool compress application
Sun protection
   Sunscreens
   Banuchi sun block mask
   Wide-brim hat or visor
Healing ointment
   Aquaphor
   Catrix-10
   Elta
   Theraplex
Semipermeable hydrogel dressings
   Flexzan
   Second Skin
   Vigilon

Oral Medications
Antibiotics (good staphylococcus and streptococcus coverage)
Antiherpetic medication
Antiinflammatory (acetaminophen, steroid)
Nonnarcotic pain medication
Sleeping medication

PATIENT INSTRUCTIONS AFTER CUTANEOUS LASER RESURFACING

You will have swelling, oozing, and crusting of the laser-treated areas of your skin for the first several days after your surgery. You must arrange *time off* from work and other social obligations during the initial healing stages (we advise a 7- to 10-day break).

Immediate Postoperative Skin Care

1. Continuously place *ice* or cool gel packs on the laser-treated skin (at least every 1 to 2 hours while awake) for the first 3 days after surgery. It is *very important* to apply ice to decrease the swelling and discomfort during the healing phase.

2. Keep your head *elevated* (in a sitting position) for the first few nights and while resting to reduce swelling.

3. In addition to icing, gently pat your healing skin every hour with a cool water compress (use a baby washcloth or another soft cloth, such as a gauze pad) while awake.

4. Gently apply a *thin layer* of the prescribed ointment with your finger tips to the treated areas every 1 to 2 hours while awake. Keeping the skin moist at all times speeds the healing process and lessens the uncomfortable, tight feeling of your skin.

5. Take all oral medications as prescribed by your physician. *Do not skip doses!*

6. Your first follow-up office visit will be scheduled within the first week after laser resurfacing (full-face resurfacing patients are seen by postoperative day 4). Additional visits within the first week will be determined based on your individual progress.

7. Continued postlaser skin care, including appropriate cleansers and moisturizers, will be individually prescribed by your physician.

8. Makeup application is provided by trained estheticians, usually within 10 days after your surgery.

9. Remember to keep your skin protected from the sun. Wear a wide-brimmed hat or the Banuci Sun Block mask when going outside.

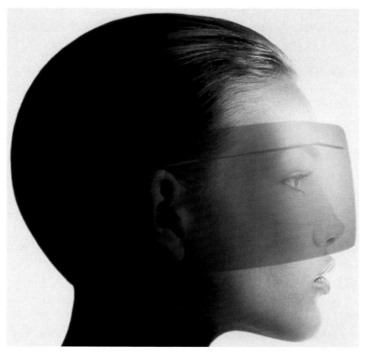

Figure 9-4

Banuchi Sun Block mask can be worn by patients postoperatively to provide 99% UVB and 95% UVA protection. Sunscreens cannot be applied to the skin until full reepithelialization has occurred. This mask or a wide-brimmed hat or visor can provide a physical block during this critical time period.

Close follow-up of all patients is necessary during the first postoperative week (Fig. 9-4). This provides an opportunity to assess the skin for infection, poor wound healing, or irritation so that early intervention can be initiated. Patients who have had extensive cutaneous resurfacing (eg, full face) may even require daily office visits to receive proper cleansing of the skin and reassurance. If the skin has been kept clean and moist during the first week and reepithelialization has been completed, makeup can be applied to camouflage the residual erythema. A nurse or esthetician who is trained in makeup application can be of great benefit to patients who need guidance with proper camouflage techniques.

After the first 7 to 10 days, patients are instructed to return every 3 to 4 weeks to track their clinical progress and to provide early intervention should any side effects or complications be encountered (see Chap. 10). Although the actual laser resurfacing procedure may only last an hour, postoperative skin care and follow-up typically continue for several months. It is thus imperative that a proper postoperative protocol be designed and implemented for all patients undergoing cutaneous laser resurfacing (Table 9-2).

CUTANEOUS LASER RESURFACING: FOLLOW-UP VISIT CHECKLIST

Postoperative day #_____

Skin appearance: _____

Evidence of infection (yes/no), poor healing (yes/no), allergy (yes/no), or

other: _____

Patient taking medications properly? (yes/no)

List medications: _____

_____

Current skin care management: _____

Patient complaints: _____

_____

In-office treatments (steam/cleanse/makeup): _____

_____

Prescribed Rx: _____

Return appointment scheduled: _____ (date)

TABLE 9–2. **CUTANEOUS LASER RESURFACING: POSTOPERATIVE DATELINE**

Postoperative Day	Skin Response	Intervention
0–7	Erythema, edema, serous discharge, crust	Daily office visits
7–10	Erythema, mild edema, no discharge or crust	Begin makeup
10–21	Decreased erythema and swelling	Begin moisturizer
21–30	Decreased erythema and swelling	Introduce glycolic, retinoic, ascorbic, azelaic acid maintenance products Look for complications
>30	Slow decrease in erythema	Monthly office visits Titrate and maximize maintenance products

Manual of Cutaneous Laser Techniques, by Tina S. Alster.
Lippincott–Raven Publishers, Philadelphia © 1997.

CHAPTER **10**

SIDE EFFECTS AND COMPLICATIONS OF LASER SURGERY

Complications of Laser Treatment of Vascular Lesions ▶
Complications of Laser Treatment of Pigmented Lesions ▶
Complications of Laser Treatment of Tattoos ▶
Complications of CO₂ Laser Resurfacing

Most cutaneous lasers subscribe to the principles of selective photothermolysis, thereby limiting energy (and heat) to the intended target rather than nonselectively and unnecessarily destroying normal surrounding skin. Nonetheless, complications can occur after cutaneous laser surgery that may be a result of technologic limitations, lack of operative skill or technique, or patient factors, such as skin pigmentation, sun exposure, predisposing medical conditions, or noncompliance with wound care.

All dermatologic lasers have virtually the same range of complications. Differences lie in the rates of their occurrence. In general, lasers that are pulsed or Q-switched (rather than continuous wave [CW] or even quasi-CW) tend to show more specificity for the intended target, whether it is vascular, pigmented, or tattooed, with less undesirable thermal damage (Table 10-1).

▶ Complications of Laser Treatment of Vascular Lesions

- ▶ Hyperpigmentation
- ▶ Hypopigmentation
- ▶ Infection
- ▶ Dermatitis
- ▶ Skin texture changes
- ▶ Scar formation

TABLE 10–1. **FREQUENCY OF COMPLICATIONS OF LASER TREATMENT**

Treatment	More → Less Complications Seen
General	Continuous wave (CW) → Quasi-CW → Pulsed
Vascular	CW argon → Quasi-CW (copper vapor, KTP, krypton, argon dye) → 585-nm pulsed dye
Pigmented	Quasi-CW (copper vapor, KTP, krypton) → 510-nm pulsed dye; QS ruby, alexandrite, YAG
Tattoo	CW CO_2 → QS ruby, alexandrite, Nd:YAG
Resurfacing	CW CO_2 → Superpulse CO_2 → High-energy, pulsed or scanned CO_2

The CW argon laser was used to treat vascular lesions in the 1970s and early 1980s, but its use was plagued with side effects, the most significant of which were hypopigmentation and hypertrophic scarring. With the development of more vascular-specific laser technology in the mid-1980s, this laser system was quickly replaced. The quasi-CW lasers, such as the copper vapor (578 nm), KTP (532 nm), krypton (578 nm), and argon-pumped dye (577 nm), are one step closer to the ultimate pulsed technology and provide good results in the treatment of telangiectasias (see Chap. 3). Side effects are usually a result of the crusting that ensues after laser irradiation, which can lead to hyperpigmentation. Transient hyperpigmentation is also the most common complication observed after 585-nm pulsed dye laser treatment (Fig. 10-1). The best treatment for hyperpigmentation is no treatment because it spontaneously resolves. Otherwise, a topical bleaching cream, such as hydroquinone, can be used to hasten the process. Other, less common side effects, such as hypopigmentation, are related to the fact that epidermal melanin overlying the targeted blood vessels can also absorb light at vascular-

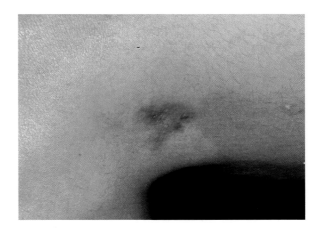

Figure 10-1

Hyperpigmentation following 585 nm pulsed dye laser treatment of leg veins shown 4 months postoperatively. Pigmentation is commonly seen using any of the vascular-specific laser systems and can last up to a year following treatment.

specific wavelengths and thus could be affected. Skin texture changes and scar formation are possible, but unlikely, events, unless excessive energy densities or overlapping laser spots are used.

▶ Complications of Laser Treatment of Pigmented Lesions

- ▶ Hyperpigmentation
- ▶ Hypopigmentation
- ▶ Infection
- ▶ Skin texture change
- ▶ Scar formation

Most pigment-specific lasers have similar complication rates. Exceptions that create more textural and pigmentary alterations due to prolonged tissue exposure times are the quasi-CW laser systems, such as the copper vapor and krypton. The quality-switched (Q-switched, or QS) ruby laser has been shown to yield more hypopigmentation postoperatively than the other QS or pulsed systems, possibly due to increased melanin absorption at the 694-nm wavelength. Overall, the most common complications seen using any of the pigment-specific lasers are related to pigmentary alterations. The use of subthreshold fluences can lead to hyperpigmentation, whereas excessive fluences can yield hypopigmentation. Other complications, such as scarring, are exceedingly rare when correct laser parameters are used (see Chap. 4).

▶ Complications of Laser Treatment of Tattoos

- ▶ Hypopigmentation
- ▶ Infection
- ▶ Skin texture change
- ▶ Darkening of tattoo (iron or titanium oxide–containing)
- ▶ Allergic reaction to released tattoo fragments

The most common complication encountered after tattoo-specific laser irradiation is hypopigmentation, which is not surprising given the fact that these same lasers are also used to target pigment. In most instances, the hypopigmentation resolves once the patient exposes the laser-irradiated area to the sun (which is not suggested during the course of treatment). Darkening of tattoo ink can be seen using any of the pulsed or Q-switched systems on cosmetic tattoos that contain iron or titanium oxide pigments (see Chap. 5). Although exceedingly rare, local and systemic allergic reactions have occurred following tattoo ink fragmentation by laser treatment. Skin texture changes can be avoided by using fluences appropriate for the tattoo type and location.

TABLE 10–2. **SIDE EFFECTS AND COMPLICATIONS OF CO_2 LASER RESURFACING**

Mild	Moderate	Severe
Prolonged erythema	Transient hyperpigmentation	Hypertrophic scar or keloid
Milia formation	Local herpes simplex virus	Ectropion
Acne flare	reactivation	Systemic bacterial or viral
	Delayed hypopigmentation	infection
	Allergy to topical cream or	
	ointment	

▶ Complications of CO_2 Laser Resurfacing

Mild
- ▶ Prolonged erythema
- ▶ Milia formation
- ▶ Acne flare

Moderate
- ▶ Transient hyperpigmentation
- ▶ Local herpes simplex virus reactivation
- ▶ Delayed hypopigmentation
- ▶ Allergy to topical treatment

Severe
- ▶ Hypertrophic scar
- ▶ Ectropion
- ▶ Systemic infection

Cutaneous laser resurfacing is associated with the highest rate of complications (Table 10-2). Although the number of reported cases of severe complications is low in the hands of experienced laser users, the incidence of these complications is on the rise as more novices use lasers.

Prolonged erythema is an expected side effect, not a complication, of cutaneous laser resurfacing and is seen in 100% of patients (Fig. 10-2). When managed properly in the delicate postoperative period (see Chap. 9), it should not lead to complications. Transient hyperpigmentation is the most common complication

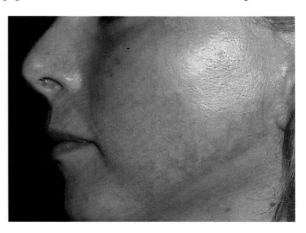

Figure 10-2
Moderate erythema 3 weeks after CO_2 laser resurfacing for atrophic scars. Note early rim of hyperpigmentation at treatment edges.

TABLE 10-3. **CO₂ LASER RESURFACING: HANDLING THE MOST COMMON COMPLICATIONS**

Complication	Intervention
Transient hyperpigmentation	Sunscreen, sun block mask
	Hydroquinone-containing creams
	Ascorbic, azelaic, retinoic, or glycolic acid cream
	Light (30%) glycolic acid peels
Herpes simplex virus reactivation	Increase antiherpetic dose
	Close skin supervision and wound care
Hypertrophic scarring	Intralesional steroid or 5-fluorouracil injections
	Silicone gel sheeting
	Pressure dressing
	585-nm pulsed dye laser treatment

seen and typically occurs in one third of all resurfacing patients. It is more frequently seen in patients with darker skin tones but can potentially occur in all types of skin. It usually becomes evident within 3 to 4 weeks postoperatively, beginning with a rim of pigmentation around the treatment borders. Patients may not realize its presence, only that it has become more difficult to camouflage the area with makeup. When left alone, the hyperpigmentation slowly resolves spontaneously, but the process can be hastened with the use of topical hydroquinone or glycolic, retinoic, azelaic, or ascorbic acid–containing creams (Table 10-3). Light (30%) glycolic acid peels can also speed the lightening process (Fig. 10-3). I usually begin peels in conjunction with a topical regimen on a biweekly to monthly basis at the first indication of hyperpigmentation to achieve the most satisfactory response in the most expeditious manner (Figs. 10-4 and 10-5).

Unlike hyperpigmentation, which is seen relatively early in the postoperative course, the appearance of hypopigmentation is delayed. It is not usually seen

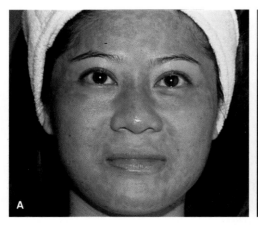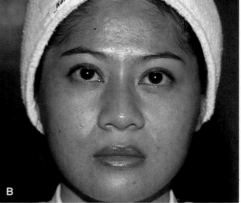

Figure 10-3
Hyperpigmented hexagonal scanner patterns noted in Asian woman 3 weeks after full face resurfacing (*A*) and again 2 weeks after a 30% glycolic acid peel (*B*).

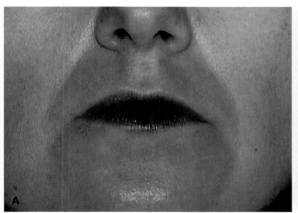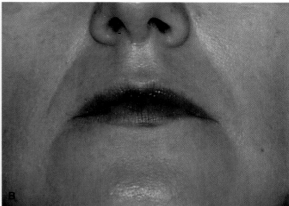

Figure 10-4

(*A*) Perioral hyperpigmentation seen 1 month after perioral resurfacing. (*B*) After two 30% glycolic acid peels and twice daily use of a hydroquinone-containing cream, the pigmentation improved.

before 6 months and may not be evident until 1 year after treatment. It is seen in all skin types, without predilection for certain areas, although it is observed more often in areas that have received a greater number of laser passes (Fig. 10-6). It is fortunate that this complication is relatively rare because its appearance may be permanent. To reduce the impact of its presence, I have been performing light (30%) glycolic acid peels of the surrounding skin. Unfortunately, exposure of these hypopigmented areas to the sun only makes their appearance more noticeable because they do not tan in a normal fashion. Reactivation of herpes labialis after perioral laser resurfacing is rare with the use of oral antiviral prophylaxis. If it does occur, the antiherpetic dose should be increased (Fig. 10-7).

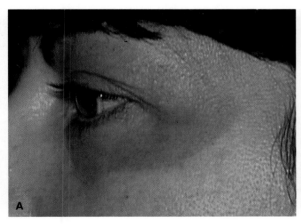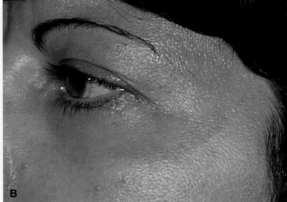

Figure 10-5

(*A*) Hyperpigmentation evident 3 weeks status-post periorbital resurfacing. (*B*) Improvement seen 4 months later with regular use of 5% glycolic and 4% hydroquinone creams.

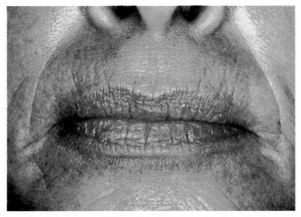

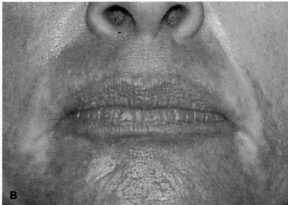

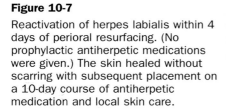

Figure 10-6

(A) Preoperative photograph of perioral rhytides. Note mild hypopigmentation at oral commissures. (B) Eight months after perioral resurfacing, hypopigmentation appeared. (Initially, hyperpigmentation was seen.)

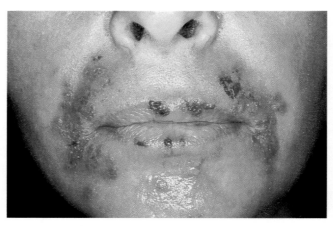

Figure 10-7

Reactivation of herpes labialis within 4 days of perioral resurfacing. (No prophylactic antiherpetic medications were given.) The skin healed without scarring with subsequent placement on a 10-day course of antiherpetic medication and local skin care.

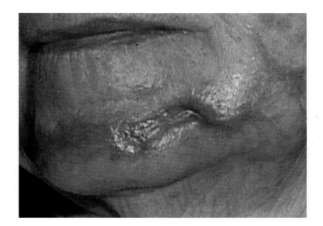

Figure 10-8

Hypertrophic scars on the chin (other scars were also present on the cheeks and forehead) which first appeared 3 to 4 weeks following full face laser resurfacing (photo obtained at 6 weeks).

The most severe complications after cutaneous laser resurfacing are scarring and ectropion formation (Figs. 10-8 to 10-10). They are rarely encountered in experienced hands, but when they occur, these complications are usually evident within the first month after the laser procedure. Intralesional corticosteroids or 5-fluorouracil can be used, as can silicone gel application, but progress is slow and scar development can continue. The use of a 585-nm pulsed dye laser typically yields immediate and significant improvement in these scars and is best implemented at the first suggestion of their appearance (Fig. 10-11; see Chap. 6). With the rising popularity of cutaneous laser resurfacing, more laser-induced scars are being seen.

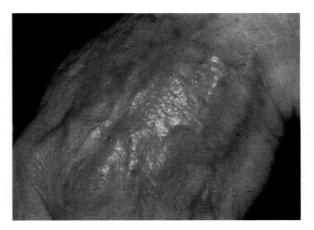

Figure 10-9

Fibrosis and hypertrophic scar formation on the dorsal hand 6 months after CO_2 laser resurfacing. Patient did not report infection or slow wound healing in the postoperative period.

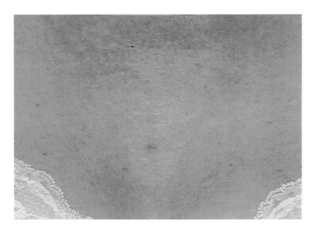

Figure 10-10

Hypopigmented areas of fibrosis on the anterior chest 12 months following laser resurfacing. Patient reported that areas were pink for several months postoperatively.

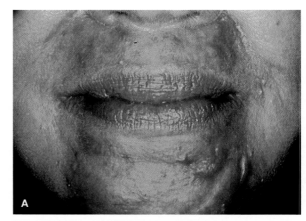

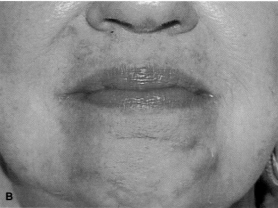

Figure 10-11

(*A*) Hypertrophic scars which appeared within the first month after perioral resurfacing, minimally responsive to intralesional corticosteroid injections (photo taken at 6 months postoperatively). (*B*) Six months later, after four treatments with the 585-nm pulsed dye laser (average fluence, 6.5 J/cm^2; 7-mm spot), scars were much improved (total time since surgery, 12 months).

► Summary

Laser technology has become so advanced that specific cutaneous targets can be eliminated without adverse sequelae to the normal overlying and surrounding skin. Despite the specificity of lasers in use today, complications can still result. Although some of these complications are laser related, most are due to operator error or postoperative mismanagement. When proper laser parameters and postoperative care are used in appropriately chosen patients, the risk of complications remains low. Using conservative laser protocols reduces the possibility of undesirable outcomes.

Manual of Cutaneous Laser Techniques, by Tina S. Alster.
Lippincott–Raven Publishers, Philadelphia © 1997.

APPENDIX **A**

DIRECTORY
OF LASER
MANUFACTURERS

Lasers

Candela Corporation
1-800-733-8550
SPTL-1B
ScleroLaser/Plus
Nd:YAG Laser
Alexandrite Laser
PLDL/Alexandrite

Coherent Inc.
1-800-635-1313
Ultrapulse 5000 CO_2 Laser
Versapulse Aesthetic Laser

Continuum Biomedical
1-800-532-1064
CB Diode/532 Pumped Q-Switched
Nd:YAG
CB Erbium/2.94 Er:YAG Laser
Medlite/755 Alexandrite Laser

Cynosure, Inc.
1-800-886-2966
PhotoGenica V
PhotoGenica T
PhotoGenica LP

ESC Medical Systems Inc.
1-800-562-5916
PhotoDerm VL

Heraeus Surgical Inc.
1-800-227-8372
Paragon CO_2 Laser

HGM Medical Laser Systems
1-800-447-0234
Digital Spectrum Series

Luxar Corporation
1-800-548-1482
NovaScan
NovaPulse

Sharplan Laser Inc.
1-800-394-2000
SilkTouch
FeatherTouch

Spectrum Medical Technologies
1-888-876-5400
Spectrum Q-switched Ruby
Spectrum CVL
Spectrum Epilaser

Thermolase
1-800-901-5562
SoftLight

Tissue Technology Inc.
1-800-658-3158
Tru-Pulse Laser

Auxiliary Equipment

Lester A. Dine Inc.
1-800-624-9103
MacroCamera

Mirror Image
1-800-841-5678
Video Computer Imaging Program

Safety Equipment

Buffalo Filter/Medtek
1-800-343-2324
Whisper smoke evacuator

Byron Medical
1-800-777-3434
Baker-David lid retractor

Oculo-Plastik
1-800-363-7004
Laser Secure Shields

Manual of Cutaneous Laser Techniques, by Tina S. Alster.
Lippincott–Raven Publishers, Philadelphia © 1997.

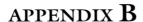

APPENDIX **B**

DIRECTORY OF LASER TREATMENT– RELATED PRODUCTS

Laser Resurfacing Postoperative Products

Banuchi
1-787-759-7490
Sun Block mask

Becton-Dickinson
1-800-267-5586
Ice packs

Beecham Laboratories
1-800-Beecham
Bactroban

Beiersdorf Inc.
1-800-537-1063
Aquaphor

Bionet
1-800-743-3795
Second Skin

Corso Enterprises Inc.
1-800-882-1056
Cold Eye Compresses

C. R. Bard Inc.
1-800-526-4930
Vigilon

Donnell DerMedex
1-800-526-3461
Catrix-10
Correction Cream Wash

Dow Hickam Pharmaceuticals
1-800-231-3052
Flexzan

Invotec International, Inc.
1-800-998-8580
Swiss Therapy Eye Mask

Medicis Inc.
1-800-716-4606
Theraplex Emollient

Swiss-American Products, Inc.
1-800-633-8872
Elta Renew

Lightening Agents

Allergan Skin Care
1-800-633-6768
Azelex (azelaic acid)

ICN Pharmaceuticals
1-800-548-5100
Eloquin Forte 4%
Viquin Forte 4%
Solaquin Forte 4%

Neostrata Company Inc.
1-800-628-9904
Neostrata lightening gel

Peter Thomas Roth
1-800-787-7526
Lightening gel (10% glycolic, 5% kojic acid, 2% hydroquinone)
30% glycolic acid gel

Maintenence Products

Allergan Skin Care
1-800-633-6768
MD Forte products (glycolic)

Cellex-C Cosmaceuticals
1-800-903-4321
Cellex-C serum/cream

Donnell DerMedex
1-800-526-3461
Catrix Correction Cream Wash

ICN Pharmaceuticals Inc.
1-800-548-5100
Glyderm products (glycolic)

Jan Marini Skin Research
1-800-347-2223
C-Esta

Ortho Pharmaceuticals Corporation
1-800-426-7762
Retin A
Renova

Makeup

Clinique
1-212-572-3829
Continuous Coverage

Estee Lauder
1-800-666-6061
Maximum Coverage Light Weight Make-Up

Sunscreens

Almay Inc.
1-800-473-8566
Almay SPF 30

Clarins USA Inc.
1-212-980-1800
Clarins SPF 25

ICN Pharmaceuticals
1-800-548-5100
Glyderm SPF 25 Sunblock

Lancome
1-800-526-2663
Lancome SPF 25 Sunblock

Penederm
1-800-395-DERM
Dura-Screen

Schering Corporation
1-908-298-4000
Shade UVA Guard/Shade 45

T/I Pharmaceuticals
1-800-782-0222
Ti-Screen

Manual of Cutaneous Laser Techniques, by Tina S. Alster.
Lippincott–Raven Publishers, Philadelphia © 1997.

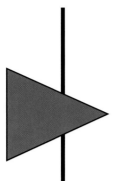

BIBLIOGRAPHY

GENERAL LASER REVIEWS

Alster TS. Cosmetic laser surgery. Adv Dermatol 1995;11:106–124.
Alster TS. Cosmetic laser surgery. In: Dzubow LM, ed. Cosmetic dermatologic surgery. Philadelphia: Lippincott-Raven, 1997 (in press).
Alster TS, Kohn SR. Dermatologic lasers: three decades of progress. Int J Dermatol 1992; 31:601–610.
Alster TS, Lewis AB. Dermatologic laser surgery: a review. Dermatol Surg 1996;22: 797–805.
Dover JS, Kilmer SL, Anderson RR. What's new in cutaneous laser surgery. J Dermatol Surg Oncol 1993;19:295–298.
Garden JM, Geronemus RG. Dermatologic laser surgery. J Dermatol Surg Oncol 1990; 16:156.
Hruza GJ, Geronemus RG, Dover JS, Arndt KA. Lasers in dermatology: 1993. Arch Dermatol 1993;129:1026–1035.
Leal-Khouri S, Hruza GJ. Aesthetic laser surgery. J Geriatr Dermatol 1995;3:249–264.
Rosenbach A, Alster TS. Cutaneous lasers: a review. Ann Plast Surg 1996;37:220–231.

BASIC LASER SCIENCE

Anderson RR. Laser-tissue interactions. In: Goldman MP, Fitzpatrick RE, eds. Cutaneous laser surgery. St Louis: Mosby, 1994:1–17.
Anderson RR, Parrish JA. The optics of human skin. J Invest Dermatol 1981;77:13–19.
Anderson RR, Parrish JA. Selective photothermolysis: precise microsurgery by selective absorption of pulsed radiation. Science 1993;22:524–527.
Dover JS, Arndt KA, Geronemus RG, et al. Understanding lasers. In: Illustrated cutaneous laser surgery: a practitioner's guide. Norwalk, CT: Appleton & Lange, 1990:1–19.
Fuller TA. Laser tissue interaction: the influence of power density. In: Baggish MS, ed. Basic and advanced laser surgery in gynecology. Norwalk, CT: Appleton-Century-Crofts, 1985.
Goldman L, Blaney DJ, Kindel DJ, et al. Effect of the laser beam on the skin. J Invest Dermatol 1963;40:121—122.
Nakagawa H, Tan OT, Parrish JA. Ultrastructural changes in human skin after exposure to a pulsed dye laser. J Invest Dermatol 1985;84:396–400.

Parrish JA, Anderson RR, Harrist T, et al. Selective thermal effects with pulsed irradiation from laser: from organ to organelle. J Invest Dermatol 1983;80:755.

585-NM PULSED DYE LASER

Alster TS. Inflammatory linear verrucous epidermal nevus: treatment with the 585 nm flashlamp-pumped pulsed dye laser. J Am Acad Dermatol 1994;31:513–514.

Alster TS. Improvement of erythematous and hypertrophic scars by the 585 nm pulsed dye laser. Ann Plast Surg 1994;32:186–190.

Alster TS. Laser treatment of hypertrophic scars. Facial Plast Surg Clin North Am 1996; 4:267–274.

Alster TS. Laser treatment of scars. In: Alster TS, Apfelberg DB, eds. Cosmetic laser surgery. New York: John Wiley & Sons, 1996:81–92.

Alster TS. Flashlamp-pumped pulsed-dye laser treatment of port-wine stains and hemangiomas. J Plast Surg Technique 1996.

Alster TS. Laser treatment of hypertrophic scars, keloids, and striae. In: Alster TS, ed. Dermatologic clinics. Philadelphia: WB Saunders, 1997 (in press).

Alster TS, Kurban AK, Grove GL, et al. Alteration of argon laser induced scars by the pulsed dye laser. Lasers Surg Med 1993;13:368–373.

Alster TS, McMeekin TO. Improvement of facial acne scars by the 585 nm flashlamp-pumped pulsed dye laser. J Am Acad Dermatol 1996;35:79–81.

Alster TS, Tan OT. Laser treatment of benign cutaneous vascular lesions. Am Fam Phys 1991;44:547–554.

Alster TS, Williams CM. Treatment of keloid sternotomy scars with the 585 nm flashlamp-pumped pulsed dye laser. Lancet 1995;345:1198–1200.

Alster TS, Wilson F. Treatment of port-wine stains with the flashlamp-pumped pulsed dye laser. Ann Plast Surg 1994;32:478–484.

Alster TS, Wilson F. Focal dermal hypoplasia (Goltz syndrome): treatment of cutaneous lesions with the 585 nm flashlamp-pumped pulsed dye laser. Arch Dermatol 1995; 131:143–144.

Ashinoff R, Geronemus RG. Treatment of a port-wine stain in a black patient with the pulsed dye laser. J Dermatol Surg Oncol 1992;18:147.

Ashinoff R, Geronemus RG. Flashlamp-pumped pulsed dye laser for port-wine stains in infancy: earlier versus later treatment. J Am Acad Dermatol 1991;24:467–472.

Ashinoff R, Geronemus RG. Failure of the flashlamp-pumped pulsed dye laser to prevent progression of deep hemangioma. Pediatr Dermatol 1993;10:77–80.

Ashinoff R, Geronemus RG. Capillary hemangiomas and treatment with the flashlamp-pumped pulsed dye laser. Arch Dermatol 1991;127:202–205.

Broska P, Martinho E, Goodman M. Comparison of the argon tunable dye laser with the flashlamp pulsed dye laser in treatment of facial telangiectasia. J Dermatol Surg Oncol 1994;20:749–754.

Dierickx C, Goldman MP, Fitzpatrick RE. Laser treatment of erythematous/hypertrophic and pigmented scars in 26 patients. Plast Reconstr Surg 1995;95:84–90.

Dover JS, Geronemus RG, Stern RS, et al. Dye laser treatment of port-wine stains: comparison of the continuous-wave dye laser with a robotized scanning device and the pulsed dye laser. J Am Acad Dermatol 1995;32:237–240.

Ellis DL. Treatment of telangiectasia macularis eruptiva perstans with the 585-nm flashlamp-pumped dye laser. Dermatol Surg 1996;22:33–37.

Epstein RH, Brummett RR, Lask GP. Incendiary potential of the flash-lamp pumped 585 nm tunable dye laser. Anesth Analg 1990;71:171.

Fitzpatrick RE, Goldman MP. Treatment of facial telangiectasia with the flashlamp-pumped dye laser. Lasers Surg Med Suppl 1991;3:70.

Fitzpatrick RE, Lowe NJ, Goldman MP, et al. Flashlamp-pumped pulsed dye laser treatment of port-wine stains. J Dermatol Surg Oncol 1994;20:743—748.

Garden JM, Bakus AD, Paller AS. Treatment of cutaneous hemangiomas by the flashlamp-pumped pulsed dye laser: prospective analysis. J Pediatr 1992;120:555—560.

Garden JM, Polla LL, Tan OT. The treatment of port wine stains by the pulsed dye laser: analysis of pulse duration and long-term therapy. Arch Dermatol 1988;124:889–896.

Garden JM, Tan OT, Parrish JA. The pulsed dye laser: its use at 577 nm wavelength, J Dermatol Surg Oncol 1987;13:134.

Garden JM, Tan OT, Polla LL. The pulsed dye laser as a modality for treating cutaneous small blood vessel disease processes. Lasers Surg Med 1986;6:259.

Garden JM, Tan OT, Ball J, et al. The pulsed dye laser for the treatment of portwine stains. J Dermatol Surg Oncol 1986;12:757.

Geronemus R. Poikiloderma of Civatte. Arch Dermatol 1990;26:547–548.

Geronemus RG. Treatment of spider telangiectases in children using the flashlamp pumped pulsed dye laser. Pediatr Dermatol 1991;8:61–63.

Glass AT, Milgraum S. Flashlamp-pumped dye laser treatment for pyogenic granuloma. Cutis 1992;49:351.

Glassberg E, Lask GP, Tan EML, et al. The flashlamp-pumped 577 nm pulsed tunable dye laser: clinical efficacy and in vitro studies. J Dermatol Surg Oncol 1988;14:1200–1208.

Glassberg E, Lask G, Rabinowitz L. Capillary hemangiomas: case study of a novel laser treatment and a review of therapeutic options. J Dermatol Surg Oncol 1989;15:1214–1223.

Goldberg DJ, Sciales CW. Pyogenic granuloma in children: treatment with the flashlamp-pumped pulsed dye laser. J Dermatol Surg Oncol 1991;17:960–962.

Goldman MP, Weiss RA, Brody HJ, et al. Treatment of facial telangiectasia with sclerotherapy, laser surgery, and/or electrodesiccation: a review. J Dermatol Surg Oncol 1993;19:889–906.

Goldman MP, Bennett RG. Treatment of telangiectasia: a review. J Am Acad Dermatol 1987;17:167–182.

Goldman MP, Fitzpatrick RE. Pulsed dye laser treatment of leg telangiectasia: with and without simultaneous sclerotherapy. J Dermatol Surg Oncol 1990;16:338–344.

Goldman MP, Fitzpatrick RE, Ruiz-Esparza J. Treatment of spider telangiectasia in children. Contemp Pediatr 1993;10:16.

Goldman MP, Fitzpatrick RE, Ruiz-Esparza J. Treatment of port-wine stains (capillary malformation) with the flashlamp-pumped pulsed dye laser. J Pediatr 1993;122:71–77.

Gonzalez E, Gange RW, Momtaz K. Treatment of telangiectases and other benign vascular lesions with the 577 nm pulsed dye laser. J Am Acad Dermatol 1992;27:220.

Greenwald J, Rosen S, Geer DE, et al. Comparative histological studies of the tunable dye (at 577 nm) laser and argon laser. J Invest Dermatol 1981;77:305–310.

Herreid PA. Pulsed dye laser treatment of telangiectatic chronic erythema of cutaneous lupuse erythematosus (letter). Arch Dermatol 1996;132:354–355.

Hoffman SJ, Walsh P, Morelli JG. Treatment of angiofibroma with the pulsed tunable dye laser. J Am Acad Dermatol 1993;29:790–791.

Kovak S, Alster TS. Comparison of a 585 nm flashlamp-pumped pulsed dye laser at normal and low fluence with a high-energy, pulsed CO_2 laser in the treatment of striae. Dermatol Surg 1997 (in press).

Landthaler M, Haina D, Waidelick W, et al. Laser therapy of venous lakes (Bean-Walsh) and telangiectasias. Plast Reconstr Surg 1984;73:78–83.

Levine VJ, Geronemus RG. Adverse effects associated with the 577 and 585 nanometer pulsed dye laser in the treatment of cutaneous vascular lesions: a study of 500 patients. J Am Acad Dermatol 1995;32:613–617.

Lowe NJ, Behr KL, Fitzpatrick R, et al. Flashlamp-pumped dye laser for rosacea-associated telangiectasia and erythema. J Dermatol Surg Oncol 1991;17:522–525.

Marchell N, Alster TS. Kaposi's sarcoma associated with acquired immunodeficiency syndrome successfully treated with 585 nm pulsed dye laser therapy. Dermatol Surg 1997 (in press).

McDaniel DH, Ash K, Zukowski M. Treatment of stretch marks with the 585-nm flashlamp-pumped pulsed dye laser. Dermatol Surg 1996;22:332–337.

Morelli JG, Tan OT, West WL, et al. Treatment of ulcerated hemangiomas with the pulsed tunable dye laser. Am J Dis Child 1991;145:1062–1064.

Morelli JG, Tan OT, Garden J. Tunable dye laser (577 nm) treatment of portwine stains. Lasers Surg Med 1986;6:94.

Morelli JG, Weston WL. Pulsed dye laser treatment of port-wine stains in children. In: Tan OT, ed. Management and treatment of benign cutaneous vascular lesions. Philadelphia: Lea & Febiger, 1992.

Mulliken JB. Treatment of hemangiomas. In: Mulliken JB, Young AE, eds. Vascular birthmarks, hemangiomas and malformations. Philadelphia: WB Saunders, 1988.

Pickering TW, van Gemert MJC. 585 nm for the laser treatment of port-wine stains: a possible mechanism (letter to the editor). Lasers Surg Med 1991;11:616.

Potozkin JR, Geronemus RG. Treatment of poikilodermatous component of the Rothmund-Thomson syndrome with the flashlamp-pumped pulsed dye laser: a case report. Pediatr Dermatol 1991;8:162–165.

Reyes BA, Geronemus R. Treatment of port-wine stains during childhood with the flashlamp-pumped pulsed dye laser. J Am Acad Dermatol 1990;23:1142–1148.

Rios WR. Flashlamp-excited dye laser: treatment of vascular cutaneous lesions. Facial Plast Surg 1989;6:167.

Ross M, Watcher MA, Goodman MM. Comparison of the flashlamp pulsed dye laser with the argon tunable dye laser with robotized handpiece for facial telangiectasia. Lasers Surg Med 1993;13:374.

Ruiz-Esparza J, Goldman MP, Fitzpatrick RE, et al. Flashlamp-pumped dye laser for treatment of telangiectasia. J Dermatol Surg Oncol 1993;19:1000–1003.

Sherwood KA, Tan OT. Treatment of a capillary hemangioma with the flashlamp pumped-dye laser. J Am Acad Dermatol 1990;22:136.

Swinehart JM. Hypertrophic scarring resulting from flashlamp pulsed dye laser surgery. J Am Acad Dermatol 1991;25:845–855.

Tan OT, Carney M, Margolis R, et al. Histologic responses of portwine stains treated by argon, carbon dioxide and dye lasers: a preliminary report. Arch Dermatol 1986;122:1016–1022.

Tan OT, Gilchrest BA. Laser therapy for selected cutaneous vascular lesions in the pediatric population: a review. Pediatrics 1988;82:652.

Tan OT, Hurwitz RM, Stafford TJ. Pulsed dye laser treatment of recalcitrant verrucae: a preliminary report. Laser Surg Med 1993;13:127–137.

Tan OT, Kurban AK. Noncongenital benign cutaneous vascular lesions: pulsed dye laser treatment. In: Tan OT, ed. Management and treatment of benign cutaneous vascular lesions. Philadelphia: Lea & Febiger, 1992:150–164.

Tan OT, Murray S, Kurban AK. Action spectrum of vascular specific injury using pulsed irradiation. J Invest Dermatol 1989;92:868–871.

Tan OT, Sherwood K, Gilchrest BA. Treatment of children with port-wine stains using the flashlamp-pulsed tunable dye laser. N Engl J Med 1989;320:416–421.

Tan OT, Stafford TJ, Murray S, et al. Histologic comparison of the pulsed dye laser and copper vapor laser effects on pig skin. Lasers Surg Med 1990;10:551.

Tan OT, Whitaker D, Garden JM, et al. Pulsed dye laser (577 nm) treatment of portwine stains: ultrastructural evidence of neovascularization and mast cell degranulation in healed lesions. J Invest Dermatol 1988;90:395–398.

Waldorf HA, Alster TS, McMillan K, et al. Effect of dynamic cooling on 585 nm pulsed dye laser treatment of port-wine stain birthmarks. Dermatol Surg 1997 (in press).

Waner M, Dinehart SM, Wilson MB, Flock ST. A comparison of copper vapor and the flashlamp-pumped pulsed dye lasers in treatment of facial telangiectasia. J Dermatol Surg Oncol 1993;19:992–998.

Webster GF, Satur N, Goldman MP, et al. Treatment of recalcitrant warts using the pulsed dye laser. Cutis 1995;56:230–232.

Weingold D, White P, Burton CS. Treatment of lymphangioma circumscriptum with tunable dye laser. Cutis 1990;45:365–366.

Wheeland RG, Applebaum J. Flashlamp-pumped pulsed dye laser treatment for poikiloderma of Civatte. J Dermatol Surg Oncol 1990;16:12–16.

ARGON TUNABLE DYE LASER

Broska P, Martinho E, Goodman M. Comparisons of the argon tunable dye laser with the flashlamp pulsed dye laser in the treatment of facial telangiectasia. J Dermatol Surg Oncol 1994;20:749–754.

Dover JS, Geronemus RG, Stern RS, et al. Dye laser treatment of port-wine stains: comparison of the continuous-wave dye laser with a robotized scanning device and the pulsed dye laser. J Am Acad Dermatol 1995;32:237–240.

Geronemus RG. Argon laser for the treatment of cutaneous lesions. Clin Dermatol 1995; 13:55–58.

McBurney E. Clinical usefulness of the argon laser for the 1990s. J Dermatol Surg Oncol 1993;19:358–362.

Occela C, Bleidl D, Rampini P, et al. Argon laser treatment of cutaneous multiple angiokeratomas. Dermatol Surg 1995;21:170–172.

Ross M, Watcher MA, Goodman MM. Comparison of the flashlamp pulsed dye laser with the argon tunable dye laser with the robotized handpiece for facial telangiectasia. Lasers Surg Med 1993;13:374–378.

Scheibner A, Wheeland RG. Argon-pumped tunable dye laser therapy for facial port-wine stain hemangiomas in adults: a new technique using small spot size and minimal power. J Dermatol Surg Oncol 1989;15:277.

Scheibner A, Wheeland RG. Use of the argon-pumped tunable dye laser for port-wine stains in children, J Dermatol Surg Oncol 1991;17:735.

Waldorf HA, Lask GP, Geronemus RG. Laser treatment of telangiectasias. In: Alster TS, Apfelberg DB, eds. Cosmetic laser surgery. New York: John Wiley & Sons, 1996: 93–103.

CONTINUOUS WAVE ARGON LASER

Achauer BM, VanderKam VM. Argon laser treatment of the face and neck: 5 years' experience. Lasers Surg Med 1987;7:495.

Achauer BM, VanderKam VM. Argon laser treatment of strawberry hemangioma in infancy. West J Med 1985;143:628.

Apfelberg DB, Greene RA, Maser MR. Results of argon laser exposure of capillary hemangiomas of infancy: preliminary report. Plast Reconstr Surg 1981;67:188.

Apfelberg DB, Kosek J, Maser MR, et al. Histology of portwine stains following argon laser treatment. Br J Plast Surg 1979;32:232–237.

Apfelberg DB, Maser MR, Lash H, et al. Preliminary results of argon and carbon dioxide laser treatment of keloid scars. Lasers Surg Med 1984;4:283–290.

Apfelberg DB, Maser MR, Lash H. Use of the argon and carbon dioxide lasers for treatment of superficial venous varicosities of the lower extremity. Lasers Surg Med 1984;4: 221–232.

Apfelberg DB, Maser MR, Lash H. Treatment of nevus araneus by means of an argon laser. J Dermatol Surg Oncol 1978;4:172–174.

Apfelberg DB, Maser MR, Lash H, et al. The argon laser for cutaneous lesions. JAMA 1981;245:2073–2075.

Apfelberg DB, Maser MR, Lash H. Review and usage of argon and carbon dioxide lasers for pediatric hemangiomas. Ann Plast Surg 1984;12:353.

Apfelberg DB, Maser MR, Lash H. Extended use of the argon laser for cutaneous lesions. Arch Dermatol 1979;115:719–721.

Apfelberg DB, Maser MR, Lash H. Expanded role of the argon laser in plastic surgery. J Dermatol Surg Oncol 1983;9:145–149.

Apfelberg DB, Maser MR, Lash H. Argon laser treatment of cutaneous vascular abnormalities. Ann Plast Surg 1978;1:14–18.

Arndt K. Treatment techniques in argon laser therapy. J Am Acad Dermatol 1984;11: 90–97.

Arndt KA. Argon laser therapy of small cutaneous vascular lesions. Arch Dermatol 1982; 118:200–224.

Brauner G, Schliftman A, Cosman B. Evaluation of argon laser surgery in children under 13 years of age. Plast Reconstr Surg 1991;87:37.

Carruth JAS, van Gemert MJC, Shakespeare PG. The argon laser in the treatment of port-wine stain birthmark. In: Tan OT, ed. Management and treatment of benign cutaneous vascular lesions. Philadelphia: Lea & Febiger, 1992.

Cosman B. Experience in the argon laser therapy of port wine stains. Plast Reconstr Surg 1980;65:119–129.

Diette KM, Bronstein BR, Parrish JA. Histologic comparison of argon and tunable dye lasers in the treatment of tattoos. J Invest Dermatol 1985;85:368–342.

Dixon JA, Huether SE, Rotering RH. Hypertrophic scarring in argon laser treatment of portwine stains. Plast Reconstr Surg 1984;73:771–780.

Dixon JA, Rotering RH, Huether SE. Patient's evaluation of argon laser therapy of port-wine stain, decorative tattoos, and essential telangiectasia. Lasers Surg Med 1984;4: 181.

Finley JL, Arndt KA, Noe J, et al. Argon laser-port-wine stain interaction. Arch Dermatol 1984;120:613–619.

Goldman L, Dreffer R, Rockwell RJ, et al. Treatment of port-wine marks by an argon laser. J Dermatol Surg Oncol 1976;2:385–388.

Greenwald J, Rosen S, Geer DE, et al. Comparative histological studies of the tunable dye (at 577 nm) laser and argon laser. J Invest Dermatol 1981;77:305–310.

Henderson DL, Cromwell TA, Mes LG. Argon and carbon dioxide laser treatment of hypertrophic and keloid scars. Lasers Surg Med 1984;3:271–277.

Hobby LW. Argon laser treatment of superficial vascular lesions in children. Lasers Surg Med 1986;6:16.

Hulsbergen-Henning JP, Roskam Y, van Gemert MJ. Treatment of keloids and hypertrophic scars with an argon laser. Lasers Surg Med 1986;6:72–75.

Janniger CK, Goldberg DJ. Angiofibromas in tuberous sclerosis: comparison of treatment by carbon dioxide and argon laser. J Dermatol Surg Oncol 1990;16:317–320.

Landthaler M, Haina D, Waidelich W, Braun-Falco O. A three year experience with the argon laser in dermato-therapy. J Dermatol Surg Oncol 1984;10:456–461.

Lyons GD, Owens RE, Mouney DF. Argon laser destruction of cutaneous telangiectatic lesions. Laryngoscope 1981;91:1322.

Maser MR, Apfelberg DB, Lash H. Argon laser treatment of cutaneous vascular lesions. West J Med 1980;133:57.

Mordon SR, Rotteleur G, Buys B, et al. Comparison study of the "point-by-point tech-nique" and the "scanning technique" for laser treatment of port-wine stain. Lasers Surg Med 1989;9:398–404.

Noe JM, Barsky SH, Geer DE, et al. Portwine stains and the response to argon laser therapy: successful treatment of the predictive role of color, age, and biopsy. Plast Reconstr Surg 1980;65:130–136.

Oshiro T, Maruyama Y. The ruby and argon lasers in the treatment of naevi. Ann Acad Med Singapore 1983;12:388–391.

Trelles MA, Verkruysse W, Pickering JW, et al. Monoline argon laser (514 nm) treatment of benign pigmented lesions with long pulse lengths. J Photochem Photobiol 1992; 16:357–360.

Wheeland RG, Bailin PL, Kantor G, et al. Treatment of adenoma sebaceum with carbon dioxide and argon laser vaporization. J Dermatol Surg Oncol 1985;11:861–864.

COPPER VAPOR LASER

Dinehart SM, Waner M, Flock S. The copper vapor laser for treatment of cutaneous vascular and pigmented lesions. J Dermatol Surg Oncol 1993;19:370–375.

Dinehart SM, Waner M. Comparison of the copper vapor and flashlamp-pulsed dye laser in the treatment of facial telangiectasia. J Am Acad Dermatol 1991;24:116.

Key JM, Waner M. Selective destruction of facial telangiectasia using a copper vapor laser. Arch Otolaryngol Head Neck Surg 1992;118:509–513.

Neumann RA, Leonhartsberger H, Bohler-Sommeregger K, et al. Results and tissue heal-ing after copper-vapour laser (at 578 nm) treatment of port wine stains and facial telangiectasias. Br J Dermatol 1993;128:306–312.

Pickering JW, Walker EP, Butler PH, et al. Copper vapor laser treatment of port-wine stains and other vascular malformations. Br J Plast Surg 1990;43:272–282.

Schliftman AB, Brauner G. The comparative tissue effects of copper vapor laser (578 nm) on vascular lesions. Laser Surg Med 1988;8:188. (Abstract)

Tan OT, Stafford TJ, Murray S, et al. Histologic comparison of the pulsed dye laser and copper vapor laser effects on pig skin. Lasers Surg Med 1990;10:551–558.

Thibault PK. Copper vapor laser and microsclerotherapy of facial telangiectases. J Dermatol Surg Oncol 1994;20:48–54.

Walker EP, Butler PH, Pickering JW, et al. Histology of port-wine stains after copper vapor laser treatment. Br J Dermatol 1989;121:217–223.

Waner M, Dinehart SM, Wilson MB, et al. A comparison of copper vapor and the flashlamp-pumped pulsed dye lasers in treatment of facial telangiectasia. J Dermatol Surg Oncol 1993;19:992–998.

Waner M, Yee Suen J, Dinehart S, et al. Laser photocoagulation of superficial proliferating hemangiomas. J Dermatol Surg Oncol 1994;20:43–46.

Wheeland RG. Copper vapor and dye laser therapy for cutaneous vascular disorders. West J Med 1989;151:650.

KRYPTON LASER

McDaniel DH, Mordon S. Hexascan: a new robotized scanning laser handpiece. Cutis 1990;45:300–305.

Waldorf HA, Lask GP, Geronemus RG. Laser treatment of telangiectasias. In: Alster TS, Apfelberg DB, eds. Cosmetic laser surgery. New York: John Wiley & Sons, 1996: 93–109.

KTP LASER

Apfelberg DB, Bailin P, Rosenberg H. Preliminary investigation of KTP/532 laser light in the treatment of hemangiomas and tattoos. Lasers Surg Med 1986;6:38–42.

Keller GS. Use of the KTP laser in cosmetic surgery. Am J Cosmetic Surg 1992;9:177–180.

Keller GS. KTP laser rhytidectomy. Facial Plast Surg Clin North Am 1993;1:153–162.

Silver BE, Livshots YL. Preliminary experience with the KTP/532 nm laser in the treatment of facial telangiectasia. Cosmetic Dermatol 1996;9:61–64.

510-NM PULSED DYE LASER

Alster TS. Treatment of benign epidermal pigmented lesions with the 510 nm pulsed dye laser: further clinical experience and treatment parameters. Lasers Surg Med Suppl 1993;5:55.

Alster TS. Complete elimination of large café-au-lait birthmarks by the 510 nm pulsed dye laser. Plast Reconstr Surg 1995;96:1660–1664.

Alster TS, Williams CM. Café-au-lait macule in type V skin: successful treatment with a 510 nm pulsed dye laser. J Am Acad Dermatol 1995;33:1042–1043.

Fitzpatrick RE, Goldman MP, Ruiz-Esparza J. Laser treatment of benign pigmented epidermal lesions using a 300 nanosecond pulse and 510 nm wavelength. J Dermatol Surg Oncol 1993;18:341–347.

Grekin RC, Shelton RM, Giesse JK, et al. 510-nm pigmented lesion dye laser: its characteristics and clinical uses. J Dermatol Surg Oncol 1993;19:380–387.

Kilmer SL, Alster TS. Laser treatment of tattoos and pigmented lesions. In: Alster TS, Apfelberg DB, eds. Cosmetic laser surgery. New York: John Wiley & Sons, 1996: 111–128.

Rosenbach A, Alster TS. Laser treatment of pigmented lesions. Geriatr Dermatol 1996; 4:195–196.

Scheepers JH, Quaba AA. Clinical experience with the PLDL-1 (pigmented lesion dye laser) in the treatment of pigmented birthmarks: a preliminary report. Br J Plast Surg 1993;46:247–251.

Yasuda Y, Tan OT, Kurban AK, et al. Electron microscopic study on black pig skin irradiated with pulsed dye laser (504 nm). Proc SPIE: Lasers Derm Tissue Welding 1991; 1422:19–26.

RUBY LASER

Achauer BM, Nelson S, Vander Kam VM, et al. Treatment of traumatic tattoos by Q-switched ruby laser. Plast Reconstr Surg 1994;93:318–323.

Ashinoff R, Geronemus RG. Q-switched ruby laser treatment of labial lentigos. J Am Acad Dermatol 1992;27:809–811.

Ashinoff R, Geronemus RG. Rapid response of traumatic and medical tattoos to treatment with the Q-switched ruby laser. Plast Reconstr Surg 1993;91:841–845.

DeCoste SD, Anderson RR. Comparison of Q-switched ruby and Q-switched Nd:YAG laser treatment of tattoos. Lasers Surg Med Suppl 1991;3:64.

Depadova-Elder SM, Milgraum SS. Q-switched ruby laser treatment of labial lentigines in Peutz-Jeghers syndrome. J Dermatol Surg Oncol 1994;20:830–832.

Dover JS, Margolis RJ, Polla LL, et al. Pigmented guinea pig skin irradiated with Q-switched ruby laser pulses. Arch Dermatol 1989;125:43–49.

Geronemus RG. Q-switched ruby laser therapy of nevus of Ota. Arch Dermatol 1992; 128:1618–1622.

Goldberg DJ. Benign pigmented lesions of the skin: treatment with the Q-switched ruby laser. J Dermatol Surg Oncol 1993;19:376–379.

Goldberg DJ, Nychay SG. Q-switched ruby laser treatment of nevus of Ota. J Dermatol Surg Oncol 1992;18:817–821.

Goldman L, Hornby P, Meyer R. Radiation from a Q-switched laser with a total output of 10 megawatts on a tattoo of a man. J Invest Dermatol 1965;44:69.

Hruza GJ, Dover JS, Flotte TJ, et al. Q-switched ruby laser irradiation of normal human skin. Arch Dermatol 1991;127:1799.

Kilmer SL, Anderson RR. Clinical use of the Q-switched ruby and the Q-switched Nd: YAG (1064 nm and 532 nm) lasers for treatment of tattoos. J Dermatol Surg Oncol 1993;19:330–338.

Kilmer SL, Lee MS, Anderson RR. Treatment of multi-colored tattoos with the frequency-doubled Q-switched Nd:YAG laser (532 nm): a dose-response study with comparison to the Q-switched ruby laser. Lasers Surg Med Suppl 1993;5:54.

Laub DR, Yules RB, Arras M, et al. Preliminary histopathological observation of Q-switched ruby laser radiation on dermal tattoo pigment in man. J Surg Res 1968; 5(8):220.

Levine VJ, Geronemus RG. Tattoo removal with the Q-switched ruby laser and the Q-switched Nd: YAG laser: a comparative study. Cutis 1995;55:295–296.

Lowe NJ, Luftman D, Sawcer D. Q-switched ruby laser: further observations on treatment of professional tattoos. J Dermatol Surg Oncol 1994;20:307–311.

Lowe NJ, Wieder JM, Sawcer D, et al. Nevus of Ota: treatment with high energy fluences of the Q-switched ruby laser. J Am Acad Dermatol 1993;29:997–1001.

Lowe NJ, Wieder JM, Shorr N, et al. Infraorbital pigmented skin: preliminary observations of laser therapy. Dermatol Surg 1995;31:767–770.

Maiman TH. Stimulated optical radiation in ruby. Nature 1960;187:483–494.

Milgraum SS, Cohen ME, Auiette MJ, et al. Treatment of blue nevi with Q-switched ruby laser. J Am Acad Dermatol 1995;32:307–310.

Nakoaka H, Ohtsuka H. Ruby laser treatment of pigmented nevi: a histologic analysis of ineffective cases. Jpn J Plast Surg 1992;35:25.

Nelson JS, Applebaum J. Treatment of superficial cutaneous lesions by melanin-specific selective photothermolysis using the Q-switched ruby laser. Ann Plast Surg 1992;29: 231–237.

Polla LL, Margolis RJ, Dover JS, et al. Melanosomes are a primary target of Q-switched ruby laser irradiation in guinea pig skin. J Invest Dermatol 1987;89:281–286.

Reid WH, McLeod PJ, Ritchie A, Ferguson-Pell M. Q-switched ruby laser treatment of black tattoos. Br J Plast Surg 1983;36:455–459.

Reid WH, Miller ID, Murphy MJ, et al. Q-switched ruby laser treatment of tattoos: a 9-year experience. Br J Plast Surg 1990;43:663–669.

Scheibner A, Kenny G, White W, Wheeland RG. A superior method of tattoo removal using the Q-switched ruby laser. J Dermatol Surg Oncol 1990;16:1091–1098.

Taylor CR, Anderson RR. Treatment of benign pigmented epidermal lesions by Q-switched ruby laser. Int J Dermatol 1993;32:908–912.

Taylor CR, Anderson RR. Ineffective treatment of melasma and postinflammatory hyper-pigmentation by Q-switched ruby laser. J Dermatol Surg Oncol 1994;20:592–597.

Taylor CR, Anderson RR, Gange W, et al. Light and electron microscopic analysis of tattoos by Q-switched ruby laser. J Invest Dermatol 1991;97:131–136.

Taylor CR, Gange RW, Dover JS, et al. Treatment of tattoos by Q-switched ruby laser. Arch Dermatol 1990;126:893–899.

Taylor CR, Flotte TJ, Gange RW, Anderson RR. Treatment of nevus of Ota by Q-switched ruby laser. J Am Acad Dermatol 1994;30:743–751.

Tse Y, Levine VJ, Ashinoff R. The removal of cutaneous pigmented lesions with the Q-switched neodymium:yttrium-aluminum-garnet laser. J Dermatol Surg Oncol 1994; 20:795–800.

Watanabe S, Takahashi H. Treatment of nevus of Ota with the Q-switched ruby laser. N Engl J Med 1994;331:1745–1750.

Yules RB, Laub DR, Honey R, et al. The effect of Q-switched ruby laser radiation on dermal tattoo pigment in man. Arch Surg 1967;95:179–180.

ALEXANDRITE LASER

Alster TS. Successful elimination of traumatic tattoos by the Q-switched alexandrite (755 nm) laser. Ann Plast Surg 1995;34:542–545.

Alster TS. Q-switched alexandrite (755 nm) laser treatment of professional and amateur tattoos. J Am Acad Dermatol 1995;33:69–73.

Alster TS, Williams CM. Treatment of nevus of Ota by the Q-switched alexandrite laser. Dermatol Surg 1995;21:592–596.

Dozier SE, Diven DG, Jones D, et al. The Q-switched alexandrite laser's effects on tattoos in guinea pigs and harvested human skin. Dermatol Surg 1995;21:237–240.

Fitzpatrick RE, Goldman MP. Tattoo removal using the alexandrite laser. Arch Dermatol 1994;130:1508–1514.

Fitzpatrick RE, Goldman MP, Ruiz-Esparza J. Use of the alexandrite laser (755 nm, 100 ns) for tattoo pigment removal in an animal model. J Am Acad Dermatol 1993;28: 745–750.

Kilmer SL, Alster TS. Laser treatment of tattoos and pigmented lesions. In: Alster TS, Apfelberg DB, eds. Cosmetic laser surgery. New York: John Wiley & Sons, 1996: 111–128.

Kovak S, Alster TS. Comparison of the Q-switched alexandrite (755 nm) and Q-switched Nd:YAG (1064 nm) lasers in the treatment of infraorbital dark circles. Dermatol Surg 1997 (in press).

Rosenbach A, Alster TS. Comparison of the Q-switched alexandrite (755 nm) and Q-switched Nd:YAG (1064 nm) lasers in the treatment of benign melanocytic nevi. Dermatol Surg 1997 (in press).

Stafford TJ, Lizek R, Boll J, Tan OT. Removal of colored tattoos with the Q-switched alexandrite laser. Plast Reconstr Surg 1995;95:313–320.

Nd:YAG LASER

Abergel RP, Dwyer RM, Meeker CA, et al. Laser treatment of keloids: a clinical trial and an in vitro study with Nd: YAG laser. Lasers Surg Med 1984;4:291–295.

Anderson RR, Margolis RJ, Watanabe S, et al. Selective photothermolysis of cutaneous pigmentation by Q-switched Nd:YAG laser pulses at 1064, 532, and 355 nm. J Invest Dermatol 1989;93:28–32.

Apfelberg DB. YAG laser meloplasty and blepharoplasty. Aesth Plast Surg (in press).

Apfelberg DB, Lane B, Marks MP. Combined (team) approach to hemangioma management: arteriography with superselective embolization plus YAG laser/sapphire tip resection. Plast Reconstr Surg 1991;88:71–82.

Apfelberg DB, Maser MR, Lash H. YAG laser resection of complicated hemangiomas of the hand and upper extremity, J Hand Surg 1990;15A:765.

Apfelberg DB, Maser MR, Lash H, White DN. Sapphire tip technology for YAG laser excisions in plastic surgery. Plast Reconstr Surg 1989;84:273–279.

Apfelberg DB, Maser MR, Lash H, White DN, Lane B, Marks MP. Benefits of contact and noncontact YAG laser for periorbital hemangiomas. Ann Plast Surg 1990;24: 397–408.

Apfelberg DB, Smith T, Lash H, et al. Preliminary report on the use of the neodymium-YAG laser in plastic surgery. Lasers Surg Med 1987;7:189–198.

DeCoste SD, Anderson RR. Comparison of Q-switched ruby and Q-switched Nd:YAG laser treatment of tattoos. Lasers Surg Med Suppl 1991;3:64.

Dixon JA, Gilbertson JJ. Argon and neodymium YAG laser therapy of dark nodular port-wine stains in older patients. Lasers Surg Med 1986;6:5–11.

Goldman L, Nath G, Schindler G, et al. High-power neodymium-YAG laser surgery. Acta Derm Venereol (Stockh) 1987;53:45–49.

Kilmer SL, Anderson RR. Clinical use of the Q-switched ruby and the Q-switched Nd:YAG (1064 nm and 532 nm) lasers for treatment of tattoos. J Dermatol Surg Oncol 1993;19:330–338.

Kilmer SL, Lee MS, Grevelink JM, et al. The Q-switched Nd:YAG laser (1064 nm) effectively treats tattoos: a controlled, dose-response study. Arch Dermatol 1993;129:971–978.

Kilmer SL, Wheeland RG, Goldberg DJ, Anderson RR. Treatment of epidermal pigmented lesions with the frequency-doubled Q-switched Nd:YAG laser: a controlled, single-impact dose response, multicenter trial. Arch Dermatol 1994;130:1515–159.

Kovak S, Alster TS. Comparison of the Q-switched alexandrite (755 nm) and Q-switched Nd:YAG (1064 nm) lasers in the treatment of infraorbital dark circles. Dermatol Surg 1997 (in press).

Landthaler M, Haina D, Brunner R, et al. Neodymium: YAG laser for vascular lesions. J Am Acad Dermatol 1986;14:107–117.

Levine VJ, Geronemus RG. Tattoo removal with the Q-switched ruby laser and the Q-switched Nd:YAG laser: a comparative study. Cutis 1995;55:295–296.

Putterman AM. Scalpel Nd:YAG laser in oculoplasty surgery. Am J Ophthalmol 1990;109:581–584.

Rosenbach A, Alster TS. Comparison of the Q-switched alexandrite (755 nm) and Q-switched Nd:YAG (1064 nm) lasers in the treatment of benign melanocytic nevi. Dermatol Surg 1997 (in press).

Rotteleur G, Mordon S, Brunetaud JM. Argon 488-415, Nd:YAG 532, and CW dye 585 lasers for port-wine stain treatment using the Hexascan. Lasers Surg Med Suppl 1991;3:68.

Shapshay SM, David LM, Zeitels S. Neodymium-YAG laser photocoagulation of hemangiomas of the head and neck. Laryngoscope 1987;97:323.

Sherman R, Rosenfeld H. Experience with the Nd:YAG laser in the treatment of keloid scars. Ann Plast Surg 1988;21:231–235.

Tse Y, Levine VJ, Ashinoff R. The removal of cutaneous pigmented lesions with the Q-switched neodymium:yttrium-aluminum-garnet laser. J Dermatol Surg Oncol 1994;20:795–800.

Yardy T, Levine VJ, McLain SA, et al. The removal of cutaneous pigmented lesions with the Q-switched neodymium-yttrium-aluminum-garnet laser: a comparative study. J Dermatol Surg Oncol 1994;20:795–800.

HIGH-ENERGY PULSED OR SCANNED CO_2 LASER

Alster TS. Comparison of two high-energy, pulsed CO_2 lasers in the treatment of periorbital rhytides. Dermatol Surg 1996;22:541–545.

Alster TS, Garg S. Treatment of facial rhytides with a high-energy pulsed carbon dioxide laser. Plast Reconstr Surg 1996;98:791–794.

Alster TS, Kauvar ANB, Geronemus RG. Histology of high-energy, pulsed CO_2 laser resurfacing. Semin Cutan Med Surg 1996;15:189–193.

Alster TS, Lewis, AB. Use of a high-energy, pulsed CO_2 laser singly and in combination with a 585 nm pulsed dye laser in the treatment of scars. Dermatol Surg 1997 (in press).

Alster TS, Rosenbach A, Huband L. Improvement of dermatochalasis with high-energy, pulsed CO_2 laser cutaneous resurfacing. Dermatol Surg 1997 (in press).

Alster TS, West TB. Ultrapulse CO_2 laser ablation of xanthelasma. J Am Acad Dermatol 1996;5:848–849.

Alster TS, West TB. Resurfacing of atrophic facial scars with a high-energy, pulsed carbon-dioxide laser. Dermatol Surg 1996;22:151–155.

Apfelberg DB, Maser MR, Lash H, White DN, Cosman B. Superpulse CO_2 laser treatment of facial syringomata. Lasers Surg Med 1987;7:533–537.

Ben-Barucg G, Fidler JP, Wessler T, et al. Comparison of wound healing between chopped mode–superpulse mode CO_2 laser and steel knife incision. Lasers Surg Med 1988;8: 596.

David LM, Lask GP, Glassberg E. Laser abrasion for cosmetic and medical treatment of facial actinic damage. Cutis 1989;43:583–587.

Felder DS, Mayl N. Periorbital carbon dioxide laser resurfacing. Semin Ophthalmol 1996; 11:201–210.

Fitzpatrick RE, Goldman MP. Advances in carbon dioxide laser surgery. Clin Dermatol 1995;13:35–47.

Fitzpatrick RE, Goldman MP, Ruiz-Esparza J. Clinical advantage of the CO_2 laser superpulsed mode: treatment of verruca vulgaris, seborrheic keratoses, lentigines, and actinic cheilitis. J Dermatol Surg Oncol 1994;20:449—456.

Fitzpatrick RE, Ruiz-Esparza J, Goldman MP. The depth of thermal necrosis using the CO_2 laser: a comparison of the superpulsed mode and conventional mode. J Dermatol Surg Oncol 1991;17:340–344.

Formica K, Alster TS. Cutaneous laser resurfacing: a nursing guide. Dermatol Nurs 1997 (in press).

Garrett AB, Dufresne RG, Ratz JL, et al. Carbon dioxide laser treatment of pitted acne scarring, J Dermatol Surg Oncol 1990;16:737.

Green HA, Domankevitz Y, Nishioka NS. Pulsed carbon dioxide laser ablation of burned skin: in vitro and in vivo analysis. Lasers Surg Med 1990;10:476.

Ho C, Nguyen Q, Lowe N, et al. Laser resurfacing in pigmented skin. Dermatol Surg 1995;21:1035–1037.

Hobbs ER, Bailin PC, Wheeland RG, Ratz JL. Superpulsed lasers: minimizing thermal damage with short duration, high irradiance pulses. J Dermatol Surg Oncol 1987; 13:955–964.

Hruza GJ. Laser skin resurfacing. Arch Dermatol 1996;132:451–455. (Editorial)

Kauvar ANB, Waldorf HA, Geronemus RG. A histopathological comparison of "char-free" carbon dioxide laser skin resurfacing. Dermatol Surg 1996;22:343–348.

Kovak S, Alster TS. Comparison of a 585 nm flashlamp-pumped pulsed dye laser at normal and low fluence with a high-energy, pulsed CO_2 laser in the treatment of striae. Dermatol Surg 1997 (in press).

Lask G, Keller G, Lowe N, Gormley D. Laser skin resurfacing with the SilkTouch flashscanner for facial rhytides. Dermatol Surg 1995;21:1021–1024.

Lewis AB, Alster TS. Laser resurfacing: persistent erythema and post-inflammatory hyperpigmentation. J Geriatr Dermatol 1996;4:75–76.

Rosenbach A, Alster TS. Multiple trichoepitheliomas successfully treated with a high-energy, pulsed carbon dioxide laser. Dermatol Surg 1997 (in press).

Waldorf HA, Kauvar AN, Geronemus RG. Skin resurfacing of fine to deep rhytides using a char-free carbon dioxide laser in 47 patients. Dermatol Surg 1995;21:940–946.

Walsh JT, Flotte TJ, Anderson RR, Deutsch TF. Pulsed CO_2 laser tissue ablation: effect of tissue type and pulse duration on thermal damage. Lasers Surg Med 1989;8:108–118.

Weinstein C, Alster TS. Skin resurfacing with high-energy, pulsed carbon dioxide lasers. In: Alster TS, Apfelberg DB, eds. Cosmetic laser surgery. New York: John Wiley & Sons, 1996:9–28.

Weinstein C. Ultrapulse carbon dioxide laser removal of periocular wrinkles in association with laser blepharoplasty. J Clin Laser Med Surg 1994;12:205–209.

Wheeland RG, McGillis ST. Cowden's disease—treatment of cutaneous lesions using carbon dioxide laser vaporization: a comparison of conventional and superpulsed techniques. J Dermatol Surg Oncol 1989;15:1055–1059.

CONTINUOUS WAVE CARBON DIOXIDE LASER

Abramson AL, DiLorenzo TP, Steinberg BM. Is papillomavirus detectable in the plume of laser-treated laryngeal papilloma? Arch Otolaryngol Head Neck Surg 1990;116:604.

Ali KM, Callari RH, Mobley DL. Resection of rhinophyma with CO_2 laser. Laryngoscope 1989;99:453.

Apfelberg DB, Druker D, Maser MR, et al. Benefits of the CO_2 laser for verruca resistant to other modalities of treatment. J Dermatol Surg Oncol 1989;15:371.

Apfelberg DB, Maser MR, Lash H, et al. Benefits of carbon dioxide laser in oral hemangioma excision. Plast Reconstr Surg 1985;75:46.

Apfelberg DB, Maser M, White D, et al. Failure of carbon dioxide laser excision of keloids. Lasers Surg Med 1989;9:382.

Apfelberg DB, Maser MR, Lash H, et al. Treatment of xanthelasma palpebrarum with the carbon dioxide laser. J Dermatol Surg Oncol 1987;13:149–151.

Apfelberg DB, Maser MR, Lash H. Review and usage of argon and carbon dioxide lasers for pediatric hemangiomas. Ann Plast Surg 1984;12:353.

Apfelberg DB, Maser MR, Lash H, et al. Preliminary results of argon and carbon dioxide laser treatment of keloid scars. Lasers Surg Med 1984;4:283–290.

Apfelberg DB, Maser MR, Lash H, et al. Comparison of the argon and carbon dioxide laser treatment of decorative tattoos: a preliminary report. Ann Plast Surg 1985;14:6–15.

Apfelberg DB, Maser MR, White DN, et al. Failure of carbon dioxide laser excision of keloids. Lasers Surg Med 1989;9:382–388.

Bailin PL, Kantor GK, Wheeland RG. Carbon dioxide laser vaporization in lymphangioma circumscriptum. J Am Acad Dermatol 1986;14:257–262.

Bailin P. Use of the CO_2 laser for non-port-wine stain cutaneous lesions. In: Arndt K, et al, eds. Cutaneous laser therapy: principles and methods. New York: John Wiley & Sons, 1983.

Bailin PL. Use of the CO_2 laser for non-PWS cutaneous lesions. In: Arndt KA, Noe JM, Rosen S, eds. Cutaneous laser therapy: principles and methods. New York: John Wiley & Sons, 1983;187–194.

Bailin PL, Ratz JL. Use of the carbon dioxide laser in dermatologic surgery. In: Ratz JL, ed. Lasers in cutaneous medicine and surgery. Chicago: Mosby, 1986.

Bailin PL, Ratz JL, Levine HL. Removal of tattoos by CO_2 laser. J Dermatol Surg Oncol 1980;6:997–1001.

Baker SS, Muenzler WS, Small RG, et al. Carbon dioxide laser blepharoplasty. Ophthalmology 1984;91:238–243.

Baldwin H, Geronemus R. Carbon dioxide laser vaporization of Zoon's balanitis: a case report, J Dermatol Surg Oncol 1989;15:491.

Bar-Am A, Shilon M, Peyser MR, et al. Treatment of male genital condylomatous lesions by carbon dioxide laser after failure of previous nonlaser methods. J Am Acad Dermatol 1991;24:87.

Bellack GS, Shapshay SM. Management of facial angiofibromas in tuberous sclerosis: use of the carbon dioxide laser. Otolaryngol Head Neck Surg 1986;94:37.

Bickley LK, Goldberg DJ. Multiple apocrine hidrocystomas treated by CO_2 laser. J Dermatol Surg Oncol 1989;15:599–602.

Blatstein LM, Finkelstein LH. Laser surgery for the treatment of squamous cell carcinoma of the penis. J Am Osteopathol Assoc 1990;90:338.

Bohigian RK, Shapshay SM, Hybels RL. Management of rhinophyma with carbon dioxide laser: Lahey Clinic experience. Lasers Surg Med 1988;8:397.

Brady SC, Blokmanis A, Jewett L. Tattoo removal with the carbon dioxide laser. Ann Plast Surg 1978;2:482.

Buecker IW, Ratz JL, Richfield DF. Histology of port-wine stain treated with carbon dioxide laser. J Am Acad Dermatol 1984;10:1014.

Buell BR, Schuller DE. Comparison of tensile strength in CO_2 laser and scalpel skin incisions. Arch Otolaryngol 1983;109:465.

David LM. The laser approach to blepharoplasty. J Dermatol Surg Oncol 1988;14:741–746.

David LM. Laser vermilion ablation for actinic cheilitis. J Dermatol Surg Oncol 1985;11:605–608.

David LM, Lask GP, Glassberg E, et al. Laser abrasion for cosmetic and medical treatment of facial actinic damage. Cutis 1989;43:583–588.

David LM, Sanders GH. Carbon dioxide laser blepharoplasty: a comparison to cold steel and electrocautery. J Dermatol Surg Oncol 1987;13:110–114.

Dover JS, Smoller BR, Stern RS, et al. Low-fluence carbon dioxide laser irradiation of lentigines. Arch Dermatol 1988;124:1219–1224.

Dufresne RG Jr, Garrett AB, Bailin PL, et al. Carbon dioxide laser treatment of chronic actinic cheilitis. J Am Acad Dermatol 1988;19:876—878.

el-Azhary R, Roenigk RK, Wang TD. Spectrum of results after treatment of rhinophyma with the carbon dioxide laser. Mayo Clin Proc 1991;66:899.

Eliezri YD, Sklar JA. Lymphangioma circumscriptum: review and evaluation of carbon dioxide laser vaporization. J Dermatol Surg Oncol 1988;14:357.

Epstein JH. Carbon dioxide laser treatment of actinic cheilitis. West J Med 1992;156:192.

Ferenczy A, Bergeron C, Richart RM. Human papillomavirus DNA in CO_2 laser-generated plume of smoke and its consequences to the surgeon. Obstet Gynecol 1990;75:114.

Garden JM, O'Banion K, Shelnitz LS, et al. Papillomavirus in the vapor of carbon dioxide laser-treated verrucae. JAMA 1988;259:1199–1202.

Garrett AB, Dufresne RG, Ratz JL, et al. Carbon dioxide laser treatment of pitted acne scarring. J Dermatol Surg Oncol 1990;16:737–740.

Goldman L, Perry E, Stefanovsky D. A flexible sealed tube transverse radio frequency excited carbon dioxide laser for dermatologic surgery. Lasers Surg Med 1983;2:317.

Greenbaum SS, Krull EA, Watnick K. Comparison of CO_2 laser and electrosurgery in the treatment of rhinophyma. J Am Acad Dermatol 1988;18:363–368.

Greenbaum S, Glogau R, Stegman S, et al. Carbon dioxide laser treatment of erythroplasia of Queyrat. J Dermatol Surg Oncol 1989;15:747.

Groot DW, Johnston PA. Carbon dioxide laser treatment of porokeratoses of Mibelli. Lasers Surg Med 1985;5:603.

Groot DW, Arlette JP, Johnston PA. Comparison of the infrared coagulator and the carbon dioxide laser in the removal of decorative tattoos. J Am Acad Dermatol 1986;15:518–522.

Haas A, Wheeland RG. Treatment of massive rhinophyma with the carbon dioxide laser. J Dermatol Surg Oncol 1990;16:645–649.

Hambley R, Hebda P, Abell E, et al. Wound healing of skin incisions produced by ultrasonically vibrating knife, scalpel, electrosurgery and carbon dioxide laser. J Dermatol Surg Oncol 1988;14:1213–1217.

Henderson DL, Cromwell TA, Mes LG. Argon and carbon dioxide laser treatment of hypertrophic and keloid scars. Lasers Surg Med 1984;3:271–277.

Hishimoto K, Rockwell JR, Epstein RA, et al. Laser wound healing compared with other surgical modalities. Burns 1973;1:13.

Huener CJ, Wheeland RG, Bailin PL, et al. Lasers: treatment of myxoid cysts with carbon dioxide laser vaporization. J Dermatol Surg Oncol 1988;29:357–369.

Janniger CK, Golberg DJ. Angiofibromas in tuberous sclerosis: comparison of treatment by carbon dioxide and argon laser. J Dermatol Surg Oncol 1990;16:317–320.

Johnson TM, Sebastien TS, Lowe L, et al. Carbon dioxide laser treatment of actinic cheilitis: clinicohistopathologic correlation to determine the optimal depth of destruction. J Am Acad Dermatol 1992;27:737.

Kantor GR, Ratz JL, Wheeland RG. Treatment of acne keloidalis nuchae with carbon dioxide laser. J Am Acad Dermatol 1986;14:263.

Kantor GR, Wheeland RG, Bailin PL, et al. Treatment of earlobe keloids with carbon dioxide laser excision: a report of 16 cases. J Dermatol Surg Oncol 1985;11:1063–1067.

Kaplan L. The CO_2 laser in plastic surgery. Lasers Surg Med 1986;6:385.

Karam F, Bauman T. Carbon dioxide treatment of chondrodermatitis nodularis helicis. Ear Nose Throat J 1988;67:757.

Keller GS. Suprafibromuscular and endoscopic rhytidectomy with the high-output carbon dioxide laser and flexible waveguide. In: Alster TS, Apfelberg DB, eds. Cosmetic laser surgery. New York: John Wiley & Sons, 1996:43–54.

Keller GS, Razum NJ, Elliott S, et al. Small incision laser lift for forehead creases and glabellar furrows. Arch Otolaryngol 1993;119:632–635.

Kirschner RA. Cutaneous plastic surgery with the CO_2 laser. Surg Clin North Am 1984;64:871.

Lanigan SW, Cotterill JA. The treatment of port wine stains with the carbon dioxide laser. Br J Dermatol 1990;123:229.

Levine H, Bailin P. Carbon dioxide laser treatment of cutaneous hemangiomas and tattoos. Arch Otolaryngol 1982;108:236.

Malek RS. Laser treatment of premalignant and malignant squamous cell lesions of the penis. Lasers Surg Med 1992;12:246.

McBurney EI, Rosen DA. Carbon dioxide laser treatment of verruca vulgaris. J Dermatol Surg Oncol 1984;10:45–48.

McBurney EI. CO_2 laser treatment of dermatologic lesions. South Med J 1978;71:795.

McElroy JA, Mehregan DA, Roenigk RK. Carbon dioxide laser vaporization of recalcitrant symptomatic plaques of Hailey-Hailey disease and Darier's disease. J Am Acad Dermatol 1990;23:893.

Mittelman HM, Apfelberg DB. Carbon dioxide laser blepharoplasty: advantages and disadvantages. Ann Plast Surg 1990;24:1–6.

Morrow DM, Morrow LB. Carbon dioxide laser blepharoplasty. J Dermatol Surg Oncol 1992;18:307–313.

Mueller TJ, Carlson BA, Lindy MP. The use of the carbon dioxide surgical laser for the treatment of verrucae. J Am Podiatr Med Assoc 1980;70:136.

Mullarky MB, Norris CW, Goldberg ID. The efficacy of the CO_2 laser in the sterilization of skin seeded with bacteria: survival at the skin surface and in the plume emission. Laryngoscope 1985;95:186.

Norris JE. The effect of carbon dioxide laser surgery on the recurrence of keloids. Plast Reconstr Surg 1991;87:44–49.

Ohshiro T. The CO_2 laser in the treatment of cavernous hemangioma of the lower lip: a case report. Lasers Surg Med 1981;1:337.

Olbricht SM. Use of the carbon dioxide laser in dermatologic surgery: a clinically relevant update for 1993. J Dermatol Surg Oncol 1993;19:364.

Ratz JL. Carbon dioxide laser treatment of balanitis xerotica obliterans. J Am Acad Dermatol 1984;10:925.

Ratz JL, Bailin PL, Lakeland RF. Carbon dioxide laser treatment of epidermal nevi. J Dermatol Surg Oncol 1986;12:567.

Reid R. Physical and surgical principles governing carbon dioxide laser surgery on the skin. Dermatol Clin 1991;9:297.

Reid R, Muller S. Tattoo removal by CO_2 laser dermabrasion. Plast Reconstr Surg 1980; 65:717–721.

Roenigk RK. CO_2 laser vaporization for treatment of rhinophyma. Mayo Clin Proc 1987; 62:676.

Roenigk RK, Ratz JL. CO_2 laser treatment of cutaneous neurofibromas. J Dermatol Surg Oncol 1987;13:187.

Ruiz-Esparza J, Goldman MP, Fitzpatrick RE. Tattoo removal with minimal scarring: the chemo-laser technique. J Dermatol Surg Oncol 1989;14:1372–1376.

Sawchuk WS, Weber PJ, Lowy DR, et al. Infectious papillomavirus in the vapor of warts treated with carbon dioxide laser or electrocoagulation: detection and protection. J Am Acad Dermatol 1989;21:41.

Schomacker HT, Walsh JT, Flotte TJ, et al. Thermal damage produced by high-irradiance continuous wave CO_2 laser cutting of tissue. Lasers Surg Med 1990;10:74.

Shapshay SM, Strong MS, Anastasi GW, et al. Removal of rhinophyma with the carbon dioxide laser. Arch Otolaryngol 1980;106:257.

Stanley RJ, Roenigk RK. Actinic cheilitis: treatment with the carbon dioxide laser. Mayo Clin Proc 1988;63:230.

Starr JC, Kilmer SL, Wheeland RG. Analysis of the carbon dioxide laser plume for simian immunodeficiency virus. J Dermatol Surg Oncol 1992;8:297.

Street ML, Roenigk RK. Recalcitrant periungual verrucae: the role of carbon dioxide laser vaporization. J Am Acad Dermatol 1990;23:115.

Taylor MB. Chondrodermatitis nodularis chronica helicis: successful treatment with the carbon dioxide laser. J Dermatol Surg Oncol 1991;17:862.

Walker NPJ, Matthews J, Newsom SWM. Possible hazards from irradiation with the carbon dioxide laser. Lasers Surg Med 1986;6:84.

Wheeland RG. Revision of full-thickness skin grafts using the carbon dioxide laser. J Dermatol Surg Oncol 1988;14:130.

Wheeland RG, Bailin PL, Ratz JL. Combined carbon dioxide laser excision and vaporization in the treatment of rhinophyma. J Dermatol Surg Oncol 1987;13:172.

Whitaker DC. Microscopically proven cure of actinic cheilitis by CO_2 laser. Lasers Surg Med 1987;7:520.

Zelickson BD, Roenigk RK. Actinic cheilitis: treatment with the carbon dioxide laser. Cancer 1990;65:1307.

VASCULAR LESIONS

Achauer BM, VanderKam VM. Argon laser treatment of strawberry hemangioma in infancy. West J Med 1985;143:628.

Alster TS. Flashlamp-pumped pulsed-dye laser treatment of port-wine stains and hemangiomas. J Plast Surg Technique 1997.

Alster TS, Allen L. Effectiveness of topical anesthesia for treatment of port-wine stains in children using the 585 nm pulsed dye laser. Lasers Surg Med Suppl 1993;5:68.

Alster TS, Tan OT. Laser treatment of benign cutaneous vascular lesions. Am Fam Phys 1991;44:547–554.

Alster TS, Wilson F. Treatment of port-wine stains with the flashlamp-pumped pulsed dye laser. Ann Plast Surg 1994;32:478–484.

Apfelberg DB, Bailin P, Rosenberg H. Preliminary investigation of KTP/532 laser light in the treatment of hemangiomas and tattoos. Lasers Surg Med 1986;6:38–42.

Apfelberg DB, Lane B, Marks MP. Combined (team) approach to hemangiomas management: arteriography with superselective embolization plus YAG laser/sapphire tip resection. Plast Reconstr Surg 1991;88:71–82.

Apfelberg DB, Maser MR, Lash H. High and low-tech solutions for massive cavernous hemangioma of the face: lasers and leeches to the rescue. Ann Plast Surg 1989;23: 341–348.

Apfelberg DB, Maser MR, Lash H. Argon laser management of cutaneous vascular deformities. West J Med 1976;124:99–101.

Apfelberg DB, Maser MR, Lash H. Treatment of nevus araneus by means of an argon laser. J Dermatol Surg Oncol 1978;4:172–174.

Apfelberg DB, Maser MR, Lash H, et al. Combination treatment for massive cavernous hemangiomas of the face. Lasers Surg Med 1990;10:217–223.

Apfelberg DB, Maser MR, Lash H. Argon laser treatment of cutaneous vascular abnormalities. Ann Plast Surg 1978;1:14–18.

Arndt KA. Argon laser therapy of small cutaneous vascular lesions. Arch Dermatol 1982; 118:200–224.

Ashinoff R, Geronemus RG. Effect of the topical anesthetic EMLA on the efficacy of pulsed dye laser treatment of port-wine stains. J Dermatol Surg Oncol 1990;16:1008.

Ashinoff R, Geronemus RG. Failure of the flashlamp-pumped pulsed dye laser to prevent progression of deep hemangioma. Pediatr Dermatol 1993;10:77–80.

Ashinoff R, Geronemus RG. Flashlamp-pumped pulsed dye laser for port-wine stains in infancy: earlier versus later treatment. J Am Acad Dermatol 1991;24:467–472.

Ashinoff R, Geronemus RG. Capillary hemangiomas and treatment with the flashlamp-pumped pulsed dye laser. Arch Dermatol 1991;127:202–205.

Ashinoff R, Geronemus RG. Treatment of a port-wine stain in a black patient with the pulsed dye laser. J Dermatol Surg Oncol 1992;18:147.

Brauner GJ, Schliftman A. Laser surgery for children. J Dermatol Surg Oncol 1987;13: 178.

Broska P, Martinho E, Goodman M. Comparisons of the argon tunable dye laser with the flashlamp pulsed dye laser in treatment of facial telangiectasia. J Dermatol Surg Oncol 1994;20:749–754.

Carruth JAS, van Gemert MJC, Shakespeare PG. The argon laser in the treatment of port-wine stain birthmark. In: Tan OT, ed. Management and treatment of benign cutaneous vascular lesions. Philadelphia: Lea & Febiger, 1992.

Chambers IR, Clark D, Bainbridge C. Automation of laser treatment of portwine stains. Phys Med Biol 1990;7:1025–1028.

Cosman B. Clinical exposure in the laser therapy of portwine stains. Lasers Surg Med 1988;3:133–152.

Cosman B. Experience in the argon laser therapy of port wine stains. Plast Reconstr Surg 1980;65:119–129.

Dinehart SM, Waner M, Flock S. The copper vapor laser for treatment of cutaneous vascular and pigmented lesions. J Dermatol Surg Oncol 1993;19:370–375.

Dinehart SM, Waner M. Comparison of the copper vapor and flashlamp-pulsed dye laser in the treatment of facial telangiectasia. J Am Acad Dermatol 1991;24:116.

Dixon J, Huether S, Rotering RH. Hypertrophic scarring in argon laser treatment of portwine stains. Plast Reconstr Surg 1984;73:771–780.

Dixon JA, Rotering RH, Huether SE. Patients' evaluation of argon laser therapy of portwine stain, decorative tattoos, and essential telangiectasia. Lasers Surg Med 1984;4: 181–190.

Dover JS, Geronemus RG, Stern RS, et al. Dye laser treatment of port-wine stains: comparison of the continuous-wave dye laser with a robotized scanning device and the pulsed dye laser. J Am Acad Dermatol 1995;32:237–240.

Ellis DL. Treatment of telangiectasia macularis eruptiva perstans with the 585-nm flashlamp-pumped dye laser. Dermatol Surg 1996;22:33–37.

Finley JL, Barsky SH, Geer DE, et al. Healing of port-wine stains after argon laser therapy. Arch Dermatol 1981;117:486.

Finley JL, Arndt KA, Noe J, et al. Argon laser–port-wine stain interaction. Arch Dermatol 1984;120:613.

Fitzpatrick RE, Lowe NJ, Goldman MP, et al. Flashlamp-pumped pulsed dye laser treatment of port-wine stains. J Dermatol Surg Oncol 1994;20:743–748.

Garden JM, Bakus AD, Paller AS. Treatment of cutaneous hemangiomas by the flashlamp-pumped pulsed dye laser: prospective analysis. J Pediatr 1992;120:555–560.

Garden JM, Polla LL, Tan OT. The treatment of port wine stains by the pulsed dye laser: analysis of pulse duration and long-term therapy. Arch Dermatol 1988;124:889–896.

Geronemus R. Treatment of spider telangiectasias in children using the flashlamp-pumped pulsed dye laser. Pediatr Dermatol 1991;8:61–63.

Geronemus R. Poikiloderma of Civatte. Arch Dermatol 1990;26:547–548.

Gilchrest BA, Rosen S, Noe JM. Chilling port-wine stains improves the response to argon laser therapy. Plast Reconstr Surg 1982;69:278–283.

Glass AT, Milgraum S. Flashlamp-pumped pulsed dye laser treatment for pyogenic granuloma. Cutis 1992;49:351–353.

Glassberg E, Lask G, Rabinowitz L. Capillary hemangiomas: case study of a novel laser treatment and a review of therapeutic options. J Dermatol Surg Oncol 1989;15:1214–1223.

Goldberg DJ, Sciales CW. Pyogenic granuloma in children: treatment with the flashlamp-pumped pulsed dye laser. J Dermatol Surg Oncol 1991;17:960–962.

Goldman L, et al. Treatment of port-wine marks by an argon laser. J Dermatol Surg Oncol 1976;2:385.

Goldman MP, Bennett RG. Treatment of telangiectasia: a review. J Am Acad Dermatol 1987;17:167–182.

Goldman MP, Fitzpatrick RE, Ruiz-Esparza J. Treatment of spider telangiectasia in children. Contemp Pediatr 1993;10:16.

Goldman MP, Fitzpatrick RE, Ruiz-Esparza J. Treatment of port-wine stains (capillary malformation) with the flashlamp-pumped pulsed dye laser. J Pediatr 1993;122:71–77.

Goldman MP, Treffer R. Laser treatment of extensive mixed cavernous hemangiomas and port wine stains. Arch Dermatol 1997;113:504–505.

Goldman MP, Weiss RA, Brody HJ, et al. Treatment of facial telangiectasia with sclerotherapy, laser surgery, and/or electrodesiccation: a review. J Dermatol Surg Oncol 1993;19:889–906.

Gonzalez E, Gange RW, Momtaz K. Treatment of telangiectasias and other benign vascular lesions with the 577 nm pulsed dye laser. J Am Acad Dermatol 1992;27:220–224.

Herreid PA. Pulsed dye laser treatment of telangiectatic chronic erythema of cutaneous lupus erythematosus. Arch Dermatol 1996;132:354–355. (Letter)

Hobby LW. Further evaluation of the potential of the argon laser in the treatment of strawberry hemangiomas. Plast Reconstr Surg 1983;71:481.

Hobby LW. Argon laser treatment of superficial vascular lesions in children. Lasers Surg Med 1986;6:16.

Hobby LW. Treatment of portwine stains and other cutaneous lesions. Contemp Surg 1981;8:21–45.

Hoffman SJ, Walsh P, Morelli JG. Treatment of angiofibroma with the pulsed tunable dye laser. J Am Acad Dermatol 1993;29:790–791.

Jackson BA, Arndt KA, Dover JS. Are all 585 nm pulsed dye lasers equivalent? J Am Acad Dermatol 1996;34:1000–1004.

Key JM, Waner M. Selective destruction of facial telangiectasia using a copper vapor laser. Arch Otolaryngol Head Neck Surg 1992;118:509–513.

Landthaler M, Haina D, Brunner R, et al. Neodymium: YAG laser for vascular lesions. J Am Acad Dermatol 1986;14:107–117.

Landthaler M, Haina D, Waidelick W, et al. Laser therapy of venous lakes (Bean-Walsh) and telangiectasias. Plast Reconstr Surg 1984;73:78.

Lanigan SW, Cotterill JA. The treatment of port-wine stains with the carbon dioxide laser. Br J Dermatol 1990;123:229.

Levine H, Bailin P. Carbon dioxide laser treatment of cutaneous hemangiomas and tattoos. Arch Otolaryngol 1982;108:236.

Levine VJ, Geronemus RG. Adverse effects associated with the 577 and 585 nanometer pulsed dye laser in the treatment of cutaneous vascular lesions: a study of 500 patients. J Am Acad Dermatol 1995;32:613–617.

Lowe NJ, Behr KL, Fitzpatrick R, et al. Flashlamp-pumped dye laser for rosacea-associated telangiectasia and erythema. J Dermatol Surg Oncol 1991;17:522-525.

Lyons GD, Owens RE, Mouney DF. Argon laser destruction of cutaneous telangiectatic lesions. Laryngoscope 1981;91:1322–1325.

Marchell N, Alster TS. Kaposi's sarcoma associated with acquired immunodeficiency syndrome successfully treated with 585nm pulsed dye laser therapy. Dermatol Surg 1997 (in press).

McDaniel DH. Cutaneous vascular disorders: advances in laser treatments. Cutis 1990; 45:339—359.

Mordon S, Beacco C, Rotteleur G, Brunstaud JM. Relation between skin surface temperature and minimal blanching during argon, Nd:YAG, and CW dye 585 laser therapy of port-wine stains. Laser Surg Med 1993;13:124–126.

Mordon SR, Rotteleur G, Buys B, et al. Comparison study of the "point-by-point technique" and the "scanning technique" for laser treatment of port-wine stain. Lasers Surg Med 1989;9:398.

Morelli JG, Tan OT, West WL, et al. Treatment of ulcerated hemangiomas with the pulsed tunable dye laser. Am J Dis Child 1991;145:1062–1065.

Morelli JG, Weston WL. Pulsed dye laser treatment of port-wine stains in children. In: Tan OT, ed. Management and treatment of benign cutaneous vascular lesions. Philadelphia: Lea & Febiger, 1992.

Mulliken JB. Treatment of hemangiomas. In: Mulliken JB, Young AE, eds. Vascular birthmarks, hemangiomas and malformations. Philadelphia: WB Saunders, 1988.

Noe JM, Barsky SH, Geer DE, et al. Portwine stains and the response to argon laser therapy: successful treatment of the predictive role of color, age, and biopsy. Plast Reconstr Surg 1980;65:130–136.

Occela C, Bleidl D, Rampini P, et al. Argon laser treatment of cutaneous multiple angiokeratomas. Dermatol Surg 1995;21:170–172.

Ohshiro T. The CO_2 laser in the treatment of cavernous hemangioma of the lower lip: a case report. Lasers Surg Med 1981;1:337.

Olsen TG, Milroy SK, Goldman L, et al. Laser surgery for blue rubber bleb nevus. Arch Dermatol 1979;115:81–82.

Pasyk KA, Argenta LC, Schelbert EB. Angiokeratoma circumscriptum: successful treatment with the argon laser. Ann Plast Surg 1988;20:183–190.

Pickering JW, Walker EP, Butler PH, et al. Copper vapor laser treatment of port-wine stains and other vascular malformations. Br J Plast Surg 1990;43:272–282.

Polla LL, Tan OT, Garden JM, et al. Tunable dye laser for the treatment of benign cutaneous vascular ectasia. Dermatologica 1987;174:11–17.

Potozkin JR, Geronemus RG. Treatment of poikilodermatous component of the Roth-mund-Thomson syndrome with the flashlamppumped pulsed dye laser: a case report. Pediatr Dermatol 1991;8:162–165.

Ratz JL, Bailin PL, Levine HL. CO_2 laser treatment of port-wine stains: a preliminary report. J Dermatol Surg Oncol 1982;8:1039.

Renfro L, Geronemus R. Anatomical differences of port wine stains in response to treatment with the pulsed dye laser. Arch Dermatol 1993;128:182.

Reyes BA, Geronemus R. Treatment of port-wine stains during childhood with the flashlamp-pumped pulsed dye laser. J Am Acad Dermatol 1990;23:1142–1148.

Rios WR. Flashlamp-excited dye laser: treatment of vascular cutaneous lesions. Facial Plast Surg 1989;6:167.

Ross M, Watcher MA, Goodman MM. Comparison of the flashlamp pulsed dye laser with the argon tunable dye laser with the robotized handpiece for facial telangiectasia. Lasers Surg Med 1993;13:374–378.

Ruiz-Esparza J, Goldman MP, Fitzpatrick RE, et al. Flashlamp-pumped dye laser for treatment of telangiectasia. J Dermatol Surg Oncol 1993;19:1000–1003.

Scheibner A, Wheeland RG. Argon-pumped tunable dye laser therapy for facial port-wine stain hemangiomas in adults—a new technique using small spot size and minimal power. J Dermatol Surg Oncol 1989;15:277.

Scheibner A, Wheeland RG. Use of the argon-pumped tunable dye laser for port-wine stains in children. J Dermatol Surg Oncol 1991;17:735–739.

Shapshay SM, David LM, Zeitels S. Neodymium-YAG laser photocoagulation of hemangiomas of the head and neck. Laryngoscope 1987;97:323.

Sherwood KA, Tan OT. Treatment of a capillary hemangioma with the flashlamp pumped dye laser. J Am Acad Dermatol 1990;22:136–137.

Swinehart JM. Hypertrophic scarring resulting from flashlamp pulsed dye laser surgery. J Am Acad Dermatol 1991;25:845–846.

Tan OT, Kurban AK. Noncongenital benign cutaneous vascular lesions: pulse dye laser treatment. In: Tan OT, ed. Management and treatment of benign cutaneous vascular lesions. Philadelphia: Lea & Febiger, 1992.

Tan OT, Morrison P, Kurban AK. 585 nm for the treatment of portwine stains. Plast Reconstr Surg 1990;86:1112–1117.

Tan OT, Sherwood K, Gilchrest BA. Treatment of children with port-wine stains using the flashlamp-pulsed tunable dye laser. N Engl J Med 1989;320:416–421.

Tan OT, Stafford TJ. Treatment of port-wine stains at 577 nm: clinical results. Med Instrum 1987;21:218–221.

Tang SV, Arndt KA, Gilchrest BA, et al. Clinical comparison of millisecond versus conventional argon laser treatment of in vivo vascular skin lesions. Lasers Surg Med 1985; 5:177.

Tappero JW, Grekin RC, Zanelli GA, et al. Pulsed-dye laser therapy for cutaneous Kaposi's sarcoma associated with acquired immunodeficiency syndrome. J Am Acad Dermatol 1992;27:526.

van Gemert MJC, Welch AJ, Amin AP. Is there an optimal treatment for port-wine stains? Lasers Surg Med 1986;6:76–83.

Waldorf HA, Alster TS, McMillan K, et al. Effect of dynamic cooling on 585 nm pulsed dye laser treatment of port-wine stain birthmarks. Dermatol Surg 1997 (in press).

Waldorf HA, Lask GP, Geronemus RG. Laser treatment of telangiectasias. In: Alster TS, Apfelberg DB, eds. Cosmetic laser surgery. New York: John Wiley & Sons, 1996: 93–103.

Waner M, Dinehart SM, Wilson MB, Flock ST. A comparison of copper vapor and the flashlamp-pumped pulsed dye lasers in treatment of facial telangiectasia. J Dermatol Surg Oncol 1993;19:992–998.

Waner M, Yee Suen J, Dinehart S, et al. Laser photocoagulation of superficial proliferating hemangiomas. J Dermatol Surg Oncol 1994;20:43–46.

Weingold D, White P, Burton CS. Treatment of lymphangioma circumscriptum with tunable dye laser. Cutis 1990;45:365—356.

Wheeland RG. Copper vapor and dye laser therapy for cutaneous vascular disorders. West J Med 1989;151:650.

Wheeland RG, Applebaum J. Flashlamp-pumped pulsed dye laser therapy for poikiloderma of Civatte. J Dermatol Surg Oncol 1990;16:12.

LEG VEINS

Apfelberg DB, Maser MR, Lash H. Use of the argon and carbon dioxide lasers for treatment of superficial venous varicosities of the lower extremity. Lasers Surg Med 1984;4:221–232.

Apfelberg DB, Smith T, Masur MR, et al. Study of three laser systems for treatment of superficial varicosities of the lower extremity. Lasers Surg Med 1987;7:219–223.

Chess C, Chess Q. Cool laser optics treatment of large telangiectasia of the lower extremities. J Dermatol Sarg Oncol 1993;19:74.

Goldman MP, Fitzpatrick RE. Pulsed-dye laser treatment of leg telangiectasia: with and without simultaneous sclerotherapy. J Dermatol Surg Oncol 1990;16:338–344.

Goldman MP. Postsclerotherapy hyperpigmentation: treatment with a flashlamp-excited pulsed dye laser. J Dermatol Surg Oncol 1992;18:417.

Goldman MP, Eckhouse S. Photothermal sclerosis of leg veins. Dermatol Surg 1996;22:323–330.

Kauvar ANB, Grossman MC, Bernstein LJ, et al. Treatment of superficial leg veins with a long pulse tunable dye laser. Dermatol Surg 1996;22:404. (Abstract)

PIGMENTED LESIONS

Alster TS. Treatment of benign epidermal pigmented lesions with the 510 nm pulsed dye laser: further clinical experience and treatment parameters. Lasers Surg Med Suppl 1993;5:55.

Alster TS. Complete elimination of large café-au-lait birthmarks by the 510 nm pulsed dye laser. Plast Reconstr Surg 1995;96:1660–1664.

Alster TS, Williams CM. Treatment of nevus of Ota by the Q-switched alexandrite laser. Dermatol Surg 1995;21:592–596.

Alster TS, Williams CM. Café-au-lait macule in type V skin: successful treatment with a 510 nm pulsed dye laser. J Am Acad Dermatol 1995;33:1042–1043.

Anderson RR, Margolis RJ, Watanabe S, et al. Selective photothermolysis of cutaneous pigmentation by Q-switched Nd:YAG laser pulses at 1064, 532, and 355 nm. J Invest Dermatol 1989;93:28–32.

Ashinoff R, Geronemus RG. Q-switched ruby laser treatment of labial lentigos. J Am Acad Dermatol 1992;27:809–811.

Dinehart SM, Waner M, Flock S. The copper vapor laser for treatment of cutaneous vascular and pigmented lesions. J Dermatol Surg Oncol 1993;19:370–375.

Depadova-Elder SM, Milgraum SS. Q-switched ruby laser treatment of labial lentigines in Peutz-Jeghers syndrome. J Dermatol Surg Oncol 1994;20:830–832.

Dover JS, Margolis RJ, Polla LL, et al. Pigmented guinea pig skin irradiated with Q-switched ruby laser pulses. Arch Dermatol 1989;125:43–49.

Dover JS, Smoller BR, Stern RS, et al. Low-fluence carbon dioxide laser irradiation of lentigines. Arch Dermatol 1988;124:1219–1224.

Fitzpatrick RE, Goldman MP, Ruiz-Esparza J. Laser treatment of benign pigmented epidermal lesions using a 300 nanosecond pulse and 510 nm wavelength. J Dermatol Surg Oncol 1993;18:341–347.

Geronemus RG. Q-switched ruby laser therapy of nevus of Ota. Arch Dermatol 1992; 128:1618–1622.

Goldberg DJ. Benign pigmented lesions of the skin: treatment with the Q-switched ruby laser. J Dermatol Surg Oncol 1993;19:376–379.

Goldberg DJ, Nychay SG. Q-switched ruby laser treatment of nevus of Ota. J Dermatol Surg Oncol 1992;18:817–821.

Grekin RC, Shelton RM, Giesse JK, et al. 510-nm pigmented lesion dye laser: its characteristics and clinical uses. J Dermatol Surg Oncol 1993;19:380–387.

Grossman MC, Anderson RR, Farinelli W, et al. Treatment of cafe au lait macules with lasers. Arch Dermatol 1995;131:1416–1420.

Kilmer SL, Wheeland RG, Goldberg DJ, Anderson RR. Treatment of epidermal pigmented lesions with the frequency-doubled Q-switched Nd:YAG laser: a controlled, single-impact dose response, multicenter trial. Arch Dermatol 1994;130:1515–1519.

Kilmer SL, Alster TS. Laser treatment of tattoos and pigmented lesions. In: Alster TS, Apfelberg DB, eds. Cosmetic laser surgery. New York: John Wiley & Sons, 1996: 111–128.

Kovak S, Alster TS. Comparison of the Q-switched alexandrite (755 nm) and Q-switched Nd:YAG (1064 nm) lasers in the treatment of infraorbital dark circles. Dermatol Surg 1997 (in press).

Lowe NJ, Wieder JM, Sawcer D, et al. Nevus of Ota: treatment with high energy fluences of the Q-switched ruby laser. J Am Acad Dermatol 1993;29:997–1001.

Lowe NJ, Wieder JM, Shorr N, et al. Infraorbital pigmented skin: preliminary observations of laser therapy. Dermatol Surg 1995;31:767–770.

Milgraum SS, Cohen ME, Auiette MJ, et al. Treatment of blue nevi with Q-switched ruby laser. J Am Acad Dermatol 1995;32:307–310.

Nakoaka H, Ohtsuka H. Ruby laser treatment of pigmented nevi: a histologic analysis of ineffective cases. Jpn J Plast Surg 1992;35:25.

Nelson JS, Applebaum J. Treatment of superficial cutaneous lesions by melanin-specific selective photothermolysis using the Q-switched ruby laser. Ann Plast Surg 1992;29: 231–237.

Oshiro T, Maruyama Y. The ruby and argon lasers in the treatment of nevi. Ann Acad Med Singapore 1983;12:388–395.

Polla LL, Margolis RJ, Dover JS, et al. Melanosomes are a primary target of Q-switched ruby laser irradiation in guinea pig skin. J Invest Dermatol 1987;89:281–286.

Rosenbach A, Alster TS. Laser treatment of pigmented lesions. Geriatr Dermatol 1996; 6:195–196.

Rosenbach A, Alster TS. Comparison of the Q-switched alexandrite (755 nm) and Q-switched Nd:YAG (1064 nm) lasers in the treatment of benign melanocytic nevi. Dermatol Surg 1997 (in press).

Scheepers JH, Quaba AA. Clinical experience with the PLDL-1 (pigmented lesion dye laser) in the treatment of pigmented birthmarks: a preliminary report. Br J Plast Surg 1993;46:247–251.

Sherwood KA. Murray S, Kurban AK, Tan OT. Effect of wavelength on cutaneous pigment using pulsed irradiation. J Invest Dermatol 1989;92:712–716.

Tan OT, Morelli JG, Kurban AK. Pulsed dye laser treatment of benign cutaneous pigmented lesions. Lasers Surg Med 1992;12:538–541.

Taylor CR, Anderson RR. Treatment of benign pigmented epidermal lesions by Q-switched ruby laser. Int J Dermatol 1993;32:908–912.

Taylor CR, Anderson RR. Ineffective treatment of melasma and postinflammatory hyperpigmentation by Q-switched ruby laser. J Dermatol Surg Oncol 1994;20:592–597.

Taylor CR, Flotte TJ, Gange RW, Anderson RR. Treatment of nevus of Ota by Q-switched ruby laser. J Am Acad Dermatol 1994;30:743–751.

Trelles MA, Verkruysse W, Pickering JW, et al. Monoline argon laser (514 nm) treatment of benign pigmented lesions with long pulse lengths. J Photochem Photobiol 1992; 16:357–360.

Tse Y, Levine VJ, Ashinoff R. The removal of cutaneous pigmented lesions with the Q-switched neodymium:yttrium-aluminum-garnet laser. J Dermatol Surg Oncol 1994; 20:795–800.

Watanabe S, Takahashi H. Treatment of nevus of Ota with the Q-switched ruby laser. N Engl J Med 1994;331:1745–1750.

Yardy T, Levine VJ, McLain SA, et al. The removal of cutaneous pigmented lesions with the Q-switched neodymium-yttrium-aluminum-garnet laser: a comparative study. J Dermatol Surg Oncol 1994;20:795–800.

TATTOOS

Achauer BM, Nelson S, Vander Kam VM, et al. Treatment of traumatic tattoos by Q-switched ruby laser. Plast Reconstr Surg 1994;93:318–323.

Alster TS. Successful elimination of traumatic tattoos by the Q-switched alexandrite (755 nm) laser. Ann Plast Surg 1995;34:542–545.

Alster TS. Q-switched alexandrite (755 nm) laser treatment of professional and amateur tattoos. J Am Acad Dermatol 1995;33:69–73.

Anderson RR, Geronemus R, Kilmer SL, et al. Cosmetic tattoo ink darkening: a complication of Q-switched and pulsed laser treatment. Arch Dermatol 1993;129:1010–1014.

Apfelberg DB, Maser MR, Lash H, et al. Comparison of the argon and carbon dioxide laser treatment of decorative tattoos: a preliminary report. Ann Plast Surg 1985;14: 6–15.

Apfelberg DB, Maser MR, Lash H. Argon laser treatment of decorative tattoos. Br J Plast Surg 1979;32:141.

Apfelberg DB, Rivers J, Maser MR, et al. Update on laser usage in treatment of decorative tattoos. Lasers Surg Med 1982;2:169.

Ashinoff R, Geronemus RG. Rapid response of traumatic and medical tattoos to treatment with the Q-switched ruby laser. Plast Reconstr Surg 1993;91:841–845.

Ashinoff R, Levine VJ, Soter NA. Allergic reactions to tattoo pigment after laser treatment. Dermatol Surg 1995;21:291–294.

Bailin PL, Ratz JR, Levine HL. Removal of tattoos by CO_2 laser. J Dermatol Surg Oncol 1980;6:997–1001.

Brady SC, Blokmanis A, Jewett L. Tattoo removal with the carbon dioxide laser. Ann Plast Surg 1978;2:482.

DeCoste SD, Anderson RR. Comparison of Q-switched ruby and Q-switched Nd:YAG laser treatment of tattoos. Lasers Surg Med Suppl 1991;3:64.

Fitzpatrick RE, Goldman MP, Ruiz-Esparza J. Use of the alexandrite laser (755 nm, 100 ns) for tattoo pigment removal in an animal model. J Am Acad Dermatol 1993;28: 745–750.

Fitzpatrick RE, Goldman MP. Tattoo removal using the alexandrite laser. Arch Dermatol 1994;130:1508–1514.

Goldman L, Hornby P, Meyer R. Radiation from a Q-switched laser with a total output of 10 megawatts on a tattoo of a man. J Invest Dermatol 1965;44:69.

Goldman L, Rockwell RJ, Meyer R, et al. Laser treatment of tattoos: a preliminary survey of three years clinical experience. JAMA 1967;201:163–166.

Groot DW, Arlette JP, Johnston PA. Comparison of the infrared coagulator and the carbon dioxide laser in the removal of decorative tattoos. J Am Acad Dermatol 1986;15: 518–522.

Kilmer SL, Alster TS. Laser treatment of tattoos and pigmented lesions. In: Alster TS, Apfelberg DB, eds. Cosmetic laser surgery. New York: John Wiley & Sons, 1996: 111–128.

Kilmer SL, Anderson RR. Clinical use of the Q-switched ruby and the Q-switched Nd: YAG (1064 nm and 532 nm) lasers for treatment of tattoos. J Dermatol Surg Oncol 1993;19:330–338.

Kilmer SL, Farinelli WF, Tearney G, et al. Use of a larger spot size for the treatment of tattoos increases clinical efficacy and decreases potential side effects. Lasers Surg Med Suppl 1994;6:51.

Kilmer SL, Lee MS, Grevelink JM, et al. The Q-switched Nd: YAG laser (1064 nm) effectively treats tattoos: a controlled, dose-response study. Arch Dermatol 1993;129: 971–978.

Levine H, Bailin P. Carbon dioxide treatment of cutaneous hemangiomas and tattoos. Arch Otolaryngol 1982;108:36.

Levine VJ, Geronemus RG. Tattoo removal with the Q-switched ruby laser and the Q-switched Nd: YAG laser: a comparative study. Cutis 1995;55:295–296.

Lowe NJ, Luftman D, Sawcer D. Q-switched ruby laser: further observations on treatment of professional tattoos. J Dermatol Surg Oncol 1994;20:307–311.

McMeekin TO, Goodwin DP. A comparison of the alexandrite laser (755 nm) with the Q-switched ruby laser (694 nm) in the treatment of tattoos. Lasers Surg Med Suppl 1993;5:43.

Reid WH, McLeod PJ, Ritchie A, et al. Q-switched ruby laser treatment of black tattoos. Br J Plast Surg 1983;36:455–459.

Reid WH, Miller ID, Murphy MJ, et al. Q-switched ruby laser treatment of tattoos: a 9-year experience. Br J Plast Surg 1990;43:663–669.

Reid R, Muller S. Tattoo removal by CO_2 laser dermabrasion. Plast Reconstr Surg 1980; 65:717—721.

Ruiz-Esparza J, Goldman MP, Fitzpatrick RE. Tattoo removal with minimal scarring: the chemo-laser technique. J Dermatol Surg Oncol 1989;14:1372–1376.

Scheibner A, Kenny G, White W, et al. A superior method of tattoo removal using the Q-switched ruby laser. J Dermatol Surg Oncol 1990;16:1091–1098.

Stafford TJ, Lizek R, Boll J, Tan OT. Removal of colored tattoos with the Q-switched alexandrite laser. Plast Reconstr Surg 1995;95:313–320.

Taylor CR, Gange RW, Dover JS, et al. Treatment of tattoos by Q-switched ruby laser. Arch Dermatol 1990;126:893—899.

Taylor CR, Anderson RR, Gange W, et al. Light and electron microscopic analysis of tattoos by Q-switched ruby laser. J Invest Dermatol 1991;97:131–136.

Yules RB, Laub DR, Honey R, et al. The effect of Q-switched ruby laser radiation on dermal tattoo pigment in man. Arch Surg 1967;95:179–180.

SCARS AND STRIAE

Abergel RP, Dwyer RM, Meeker CA, et al. Laser treatment of keloids: a clinical trial and an in vitro study with Nd: YAG laser. Lasers Surg Med 1984;4:291–295.

Alster TS. Improvement of erythematous and hypertrophic scars by the 585 nm pulsed dye laser. Ann Plast Surg 1994;32:186–190.

Alster TS. Laser treatment of erythematous/hypertrophic and pigmented scars in 26 patients: a discussion. Plast Reconstr Surg 1995;95:91–92.

Alster TS. Laser treatment of hypertrophic scars. Facial Plast Surg Clin North Am 1996; 4:267–274.

Alster TS. Laser treatment of scars. In: Alster TS, Apfelberg DB, eds. Cosmetic laser surgery. New York: John Wiley & Sons, 1996:81–92.

Alster TS. Laser treatment of hypertrophic scars, keloids, and striae. In: Alster TS, ed. Dermatologic clinics. Philadelphia: WB Saunders, 1997 (in press).

Alster TS, Kurban AK, Grove GL, et al. Alteration of argon laser-induced scars by the pulsed dye laser. Lasers Surg Med 1993;13:368–373.

Alster TS, Lewis AB. Use of a high-energy, pulsed CO_2 laser singly and in combination with a 585 nm pulsed dye laser in the treatment of scars. Dermatol Surg 1997 (in press).

Alster TS, McMeekin TO. Improvement of facial acne scars by the 585 nm flashlamp-pumped dye laser. J Am Acad Dermatol 1996;35:79–81.

Alster TS, West TB. Resurfacing of atrophic facial scars with a high-energy, pulsed carbon-dioxide laser. Dermatol Surg 1996;22:151–155.

Alster TS, Williams CM. Treatment of keloid sternotomy scars with the 585 nm flashlamp-pumped pulsed dye laser. Lancet 1995;345:1198–1200.

Apfelberg DB, Maser MR, Lash H, et al. Preliminary results of argon and carbon dioxide laser treatment of keloid scars. Lasers Surg Med 1984;4:283–290.

Apfelberg DB, Maser MR, White DN, Lash H. Failure of carbon dioxide laser excision of keloids. Lasers Surg Med 1989;9:382–388.

Dierickx C, Goldman MP, Fitzpatrick RE. Laser treatment of erythematous/hypertrophic and pigmented scars in 26 patients. Plast Reconstr Surg 1995;95:84–90.

Henderson DL, Cromwell TA, Mes LG. Argon and carbon dioxide laser treatment of hypertrophic and keloid scars. Lasers Surg Med 1984;3:271–277.

Hulsbergen-Henning JP, Roskam Y, van Gemert MJ. Treatment of keloids and hypertrophic scars with an argon laser. Lasers Surg Med 1986;6:72–75.

Kantor GR, Wheeland RG, Bailin PL, et al. Treatment of earlobe keloids with carbon dioxide laser excision: a report of 16 cases. J Dermatol Surg Oncol 1985;11:1063–1067.

Kovak S, Alster TS. Comparison of a 585nm flashlamp-pumped pulsed dye laser at normal and low fluence with a high-energy, pulsed CO_2 laser in the treatment of striae. Dermatol Surg 1997 (in press).

Lim TC, Tan OT. Carbon dioxide laser for keloids. Plast Reconstr Surg 1991;88:1111.

McDaniel DH, Ash K, Zukowski M. Treatment of stretch marks with the 585-nm flashlamp-pumped pulsed dye laser. Dermatol Surg 1996;22:332–337.

Norris JE. The effect of carbon dioxide laser surgery on the recurrence of keloids. Plast Reconstr Surg 1991;87:44–49.

Sherman R, Rosenfeld H. Experience with the Nd:YAG laser in the treatment of keloid scars. Ann Plast Surg 1988;21:231–235.

Stern JC, Lucente FE. Carbon dioxide laser excision of earlobe keloids: a prospective study and critical analysis of existing data. Arch Otolaryngol Head Neck Surg 1989;115:1107–1111.

West TB. Laser resurfacing of atrophic scars. Dermatol Clin 1997 (in press).

LASER RESURFACING

Alster TS. Comparison of two high-energy, pulsed CO_2 lasers in the treatment of periorbital rhytides. Dermatol Surg 1996;22:541–545.

Alster TS, Garg S. Treatment of facial rhytides with a high-energy, pulsed carbon dioxide laser. Plast Reconstr Surg 1996;98:791–794.

Alster TS, Kauvar ANB, Geronemus RG. Histology of high-energy, pulsed CO_2 laser resurfacing. Semin Cutan Med Surg 1996;15:189–193.

Alster TS, Rosenbach A, Huband L. Improvement of dermatochalasis with high-energy, pulsed CO_2 laser cutaneous resurfacing. Dermatol Surg 1997 (in press).

Alster TS, West TB. Resurfacing of atrophic facial scars with a high-energy pulsed carbon dioxide laser. Dermatol Surg 1996;22:151–155.

David LM, Lask GP, Glassberg E. Laser abrasion for cosmetic and medical treatment of facial actinic damage. Cutis 1989;43:583–587.

Dover JS. CO_2 laser resurfacing: why all the fuss? Plast Reconstr Surg 1996;98:506–509.

Felder DS, Mayl N. Periorbital carbon dioxide laser resurfacing. Semin Ophthalmol 1996; 11:201–210.

Fitzpatrick RE, Goldman MP. Advances in carbon dioxide laser surgery. Clin Dermatol 1995;13:35–47.

Fitzpatrick RE, Goldman MP, Satur N, Tope WD. Pulsed CO_2 resurfacing of photodamaged facial skin. Arch Dermatol 1996;132:395.

Formica K, Alster TS. Cutaneous laser resurfacing: a nursing guide. Dermatol Nurs 1997.

Ho C, Nguyen Q, Lowe N, et al. Laser resurfacing in pigmented skin. Dermatol Surg 1995;21:1035–1037.

Hruza GJ. Laser skin resurfacing. Arch Dermatol 1996;132:451–455. (Editorial)

Kauvar ANB, Waldorf HA, Geronemus RG. A histopathological comparison of "char-free" carbon dioxide laser skin resurfacing. Dermatol Surg 1996;22:343–348.

Lask G, Keller G, Lowe N, Gormley D. Laser skin resurfacing with the SilkTouch Flashscanner for facial rhytides. Dermatol Surg 1995;21:1021–1024.

Lewis AB, Alster TS. Laser resurfacing: persistent erythema and post-inflammatory hyperpigmentation. J Geriatr Dermatol 1996;4:75–76.

Lowe NJ, Lask G, Griffin ME, et al. Skin resurfacing with the Ultrapulse carbon dioxide laser. Dermatol Surg 1995;21:1025.

Waldorf HA, Kauvar AN, Geronemus RG. Skin resurfacing of fine to deep rhytides using a char-free carbon dioxide laser in 47 patients. Dermatol Surg 1995;21:940–946.

Weinstein C. Ultrapulse carbon dioxide laser removal of periocular wrinkles in association with laser blepharoplasty. J Clin Laser Med Surg 1994;12:205–209.

Weinstein C, Alster TS. Skin resurfacing with high-energy, pulsed carbon dioxide lasers. In: Alster TS, Apfelberg DB, eds. Cosmetic laser surgery. New York: John Wiley & Sons, 1996:9–28.

West TB. Laser resurfacing of atrophic scars. Dermatol Clin 1997 (in press).

LASER BLEPHAROPLASTY

Apfelberg DB. Laser-assisted blepharoplasty and meloplasty. In: Alster TS, Apfelberg DB, eds. Cosmetic laser surgery. New York: John Wiley & Sons, 1996:29–41.

Apfelberg D. YAG laser meloplasty and blepharoplasty. Aesth Plast Surg 1995;19: 231–235.

Baker SS. Carbon dioxide laser upper lid blepharoplasty. Am J Cosmetic Surg 1992;9: 141–145.

Baker SS, Muenzler WS, Small RG, et al. Carbon dioxide laser blepharoplasty. Ophthalmology 1984;91:238–243.

Beeson WM, Kabaker S, Keller GS. Carbon dioxide laser blepharoplasty: a comparison to electrosurgery. Int J Aesth Restor Surg 1994;2:33–36.

David LM. The laser approach to blepharoplasty. J Dermatol Surg Oncol 1988;14: 741–746.

David LM, Sanders G. Carbon dioxide laser blepharoplasty: a comparison to cold steel and electro-cautery. J Dermatol Surg Oncol 1987;13:110–114.

Keller GS, Cray J. Laser-assisted surgery of the aging face. Facial Plast Surg Clin North Am 1995;3:319–341.

Mittelman HM, Apfelberg DB. Carbon dioxide laser blepharoplasty: advantages and disadvantages. Ann Plast Surg 1990;24:1–6.

Morrow DM, Morrow LB. Carbon dioxide laser blepharoplasty: a comparison with cold-steel surgery. J Dermatol Surg Oncol 1992;18:307–313.

Putterman AM. Scalpel Nd:YAG laser in oculoplasty surgery. Am J Ophthalmol 1990; 109:581–584.

Trelles MA, Sanchez J, Sala P, et al. Surgical removal of lower eyelid fat using the carbon dioxide laser. Am J Cosmetic Surg 1992;9:149–152.

Weinstein C. Ultrapulse carbon dioxide laser removal of periocular wrinkles in association with laser blepharoplasty. J Clin Laser Med Surg 1994;12:205–209.

LASER HAIR REMOVAL

Goldberg DJ. Topical solution assisted laser hair removal. Lasers Surg Med 1995;S7:47.

Grossman MC, Diericky C, Farinelli W, et al. Damage to hair follicles by normal-mode ruby laser pulses. J Am Acad Dermatol 1996;35:889–894.

LASER HAIR TRANSPLANTATION

Unger WP. Laser hair transplantation. J Dermatol Surg Oncol 1994;20:515–521.

Unger WP. Laser hair transplantation II. Dermatol Surg 1995;21:759–765.

Unger WP. Laser hair transplantation. In: Alster TS, Apfelberg DB, eds. Cosmetic laser surgery. New York: John Wiley & Sons, 1996:55–66.

Unger WP, David LM. Laser hair transplantation. J Dermatol Surg Oncol 1994;20: 515–521.

MISCELLANEOUS

Alster TS. Inflammatory linear verrucous epidermal nevus: treatment with the 585 nm flashlamp-pumped pulsed dye laser. J Am Acad Dermatol 1994;31:513–514.

Alster TS, West TB. Ultrapulse CO_2 laser ablation of xanthelasma. J Am Acad Dermatol 1996;34:848–849.

Alster TS, Wilson F. Focal dermal hypoplasia (Goltz syndrome): treatment of cutaneous lesions with the 585 nm flashlamp-pumped pulsed dye laser. Arch Dermatol 1995; 131:143–144.

Apfelberg DB, Druker D, Maser MR, et al: Benefits of the CO_2 laser for verruca resistant to other modalities of treatment. J Dermatol Surg Oncol 1989;15:371.

Apfelberg DB, Maser MR, Lash H, White DN, Cosman B. Superpulse CO_2 laser treatment of facial syringomata. Lasers Surg Med 1987;7:533–537.

Apfelberg DB, Maser MR, Lash H, et al. Treatment of xanthelasma palpebrarum with the carbon dioxide laser. J Dermatol Surg Oncol 1987;13:149–151.

Baggish MS, Poiesz BJ, Joret D, et al. Presence of human immunodeficiency virus DNA in laser smoke. Lasers Surg Med 1991;11:197.

Baldwin H, Geronemus R. Carbon dioxide laser vaporization of Zoon's balanitis: a case report. J Dermatol Surg Oncol 1989;15:491.

Bellack GS, Shapshay SM. Management of facial angiofibromas in tuberous sclerosis: use of the carbon dioxide laser. Otolaryngol Head Neck Surg 1986;94:37.

Bickley LK, Goldberg DJ. Multiple apocrine hidrocystomas treated by CO_2 laser. J Dermatol Surg Oncol 1989;15:599–602.

David LM. Laser vermilion ablation for actinic chelitis. J Dermatol Surg Oncol 1985;11: 605–608.

Dufresne RG Jr, Garrett AB, Bailin PL, Ratz JL. Carbon dioxide laser treatment of chronic actinic cheilitis. J Am Acad Dermatol 1988;19:876–878.

Ellis DL. Treatment of telangiectasia macularis eruptiva perstans with the 585-nm flashlamp-pumped dye laser. Dermatol Surg 1996;22:33–37.

Garden JM, O'Banion K, Shelnitz LS, et al. Papillomavirus in the vapor of carbon dioxide laser-treated verrucae. JAMA 1988;259:1199–1202.

Greenbaum S, Glogau R, Stegman S, et al. Carbon dioxide laser treatment of erythroplasia of Queyrat. J Dermatol Surg Oncol 1989;15:747.

Greenbaum SS, Krull EA, Watnick K. Comparison of CO_2 laser and electrosurgery in the treatment of rhinophyma. J Am Acad Dermatol 1988;18:363–368.

Groot DW, Johnston PA. Carbon dioxide laser treatment of porokeratoses of Mibelli. Lasers Surg Med 1985;5:603.

Haas A, Wheeland RG. Treatment of massive rhinophyma with the carbon dioxide laser. J Dermatol Surg Oncol 1990;16:645–649.

Hohenleutner U, Landthaler M. Laser therapy of verrucous epidermal nevi. Clin Exp Dermatol 1993;18:124–127.

Huener CJ, Wheeland RG, Bailin PL, et al. Lasers: treatment of myxoid cysts with carbon dioxide laser vaporization. J Dermatol Surg Oncol 1988;29:357–369.

Janniger CK, Golberg DJ. Angiofibromas in tuberous sclerosis: comparison of treatment by carbon dioxide and argon laser. J Dermatol Surg Oncol 1990;16:317–320.

Karam F, Bauman T. Carbon dioxide treatment of chondrodermatitis nodularis helicis. Ear Nose Throat J 1988;67:757.

McBurney EI, Rosen DA. Carbon dioxide laser treatment of verruca vulgaris. J Dermatol Surg Oncol 1984;10:45–48.

McDaniel DH, Ash K, Zukowski M. Treatment of stretch marks with the 585-nm flashlamp-pumped pulsed dye laser. Dermatol Surg 1996;22:332–337.

McElroy JA, Mehregan DA, Roenigk RK. Carbon dioxide laser vaporization of recalcitrant symptomatic plaques of Hailey-Hailey disease and Darier's disease, J Am Acad Dermatol 1990;23:893.

Mueller TJ, Carlson BA, Lindy MP. The use of the carbon dioxide surgical laser for the treatment of verrucae. J Am Podiatr Med Assoc 1980;70:136.

Potozkin JR, Geronemus RG. Treatment of poikilodermatous component of the Rothmund-Thomson syndrome with the flashlamp-pumped pulsed dye laser: a case report. Pediatr Dermatol 1991;8:162–165.

Rabbin PE, Baldwin HE. Treatment of porokeratoses of Mibelli with CO_2 laser vaporization versus surgical excision with split-thickness skin graft. J Dermatol Surg Oncol 1993;19:199.

Ratz JL. Carbon dioxide laser treatment of balanitis xerotica obliterans. J Am Acad Dermatol 1984;10:925.

Ratz JL, Bailin PL, Lakeland RF. Carbon dioxide laser treatment of epidermal nevi. J Dermatol Surg Oncol 1986;12:567–570.

Roenigk RK, Ratz JL. CO_2 laser treatment of cutaneous neurofibromas. J Dermatol Surg Oncol 1987;13:187–190.

Rosenbach A, Alster TS. Multiple trichoepitheliomas successfully treated with a high-energy, pulsed carbon dioxide laser. Dermatol Surg 1997 (in press).

Sawchuk WS, Weber PJ, Lowy DR, et al. Infectious papillomavirus in the vapor of warts treated with carbon dioxide laser or electrocoagulation: detection and protection. J Am Acad Dermatol 1989;21:41.

Shapshay SM, Strong MS, Anastasi GW, et al. Removal of rhinophyma with the carbon dioxide laser: a preliminary report. Arch Otolaryngol 1980;106:257–259.

Spenler CW, Achauer BM, Vander Kam VM. Treatment of extensive adenoma sebaceum with a carbon dioxide laser. Ann Plast Surg 1988;20:586–589.

Stanley RJ, Roenigk RK. Actinic cheilitis: treatment with the carbon dioxide laser. Mayo Clin Proc 1988;63:230–235.

Street ML, Roenigk RK. Recalcitrant periungual verrucae: the role of carbon dioxide laser vaporization. J Am Acad Dermatol 1990;23:115.

Tan OT, Hurwitz RM, Stafford TJ. Pulsed dye laser treatment of recalcitrant verrucae: a preliminary report. Laser Surg Med 1993;13:127–137.

Taylor MB. Chondrodermatitis nodularis chronica helicis: successful treatment with the carbon dioxide laser. J Dermatol Surg Oncol 1991;17:862.

Webster GF, Satur N, Goldman MP, et al. Treatment of recalcitrant warts using the pulsed dye laser. Cutis 1995;56:230–232.

Weingold D, White P, Burton CS. Treatment of lymphangioma circumscriptum with tunable dye laser. Cutis 1990;45:365–356.

Weston J, Apfelberg DB, Maser MR, et al. Carbon dioxide laserbrasion for treatment of adenoma sebaceum in tuberous sclerosis. Ann Plast Surg 1985;15:132–137.

Wheeland RG, Applebaum J. Flashlamp-pumped pulsed dye laser therapy for poikiloderma of Civatte. J Dermatol Surg Oncol 1990;16:12.

Wheeland RG, Bailin PL, Kantor G, et al. Treatment of adenoma sebaceum with carbon dioxide and argon laser vaporization. J Dermatol Surg Oncol 1985;11:861–864.

Wheeland RG, Bailin PL, Kronberg E. Carbon dioxide (CO_2) laser vaporization for the treatment of trichoepitheliomata. J Dermatol Surg Oncol 1984;10:470–474.

Wheeland RG, Bailin PL, Ratz JL. Combined carbon dioxide laser excision and vaporization in the treatment of rhinophyma. J Dermatol Surg Oncol 1987;13:172–177.

Wheeland RG, Bailin PL, Reynolds O, et al. Carbon dioxide (CO_2) laser vaporization of multiple facial syringomas. J Dermatol Surg Oncol 1986;12:223–228.

Wheeland RG, McGillis ST. Cowden's disease: treatment of cutaneous lesions using carbon dioxide laser vaporization. A comparison of conventional and superpulsed techniques. J Dermatol Surg Oncol 1989;15:1055–1059.

INDEX

Page numbers followed by *f* indicate figures; *t* following a page number indicates tabular material.